P9-BYE-415

# TOTAL FITNESS

*An Advanced Training Guide*
*for the Sportsperson*

| Ainsworh | CALL No. 613.711 MAR |
|---|---|
| 251112 | |
| 29.4.11 | 36.95 |
| / H | ℗ |
| ...ELD MUNICIPAL COUNCIL | |

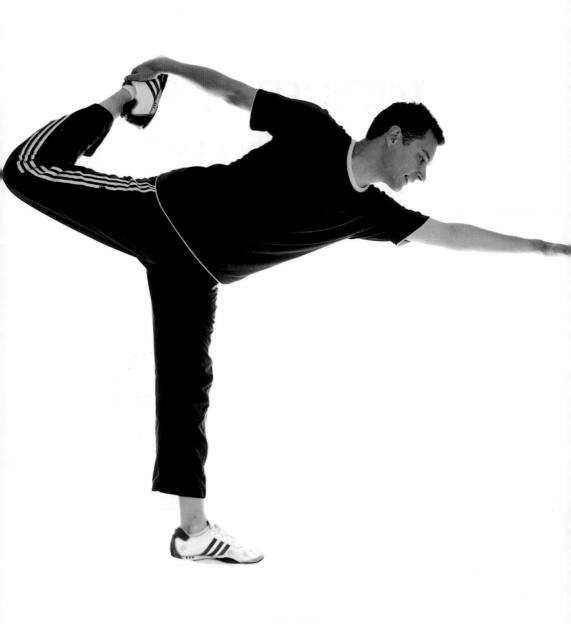

# TOTAL FITNESS

## An Advanced Training Guide for the Sportsperson

### Nita A. Martin

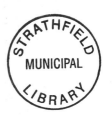

STRATHFIELD MUNICIPAL LIBRARY

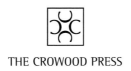

THE CROWOOD PRESS

First published in 2010 by
The Crowood Press Ltd
Ramsbury, Marlborough
Wiltshire SN8 2HR

**www.crowood.com**

© Nita A. Martin 2010

All rights reserved. No part of this publication may be reproduced or
transmitted in any form or by any means, electronic or mechanical, including
photocopy, recording, or any information storage and retrieval system,
without permission in writing from the publishers.

**British Library Cataloguing-in-Publication Data**
A catalogue record for this book is available from the British Library.

ISBN 978 1 84797 186 9

**Disclaimer**
Whilst every effort has been made to ensure that the content of this book is
as technically accurate as possible, neither the author nor the publishers can
accept responsibility for any injury or loss sustained as a result of the use of
this material. It is the responsibility of the individual to ensure that they are
fit to participate and they should seek medical advice from a qualified
professional where appropriate.

**Acknowledgements**
Thanks to Ashley Martin for taking part in the photo shoot and to Kevin
Wood for the photography.

Designed and typeset by Focus Publishing,
11a St Botolph's Road, Sevenoaks, Kent TN13 3AJ

Printed and bound in Malaysia by Times Offset (M) Sdn Bhd

# Contents

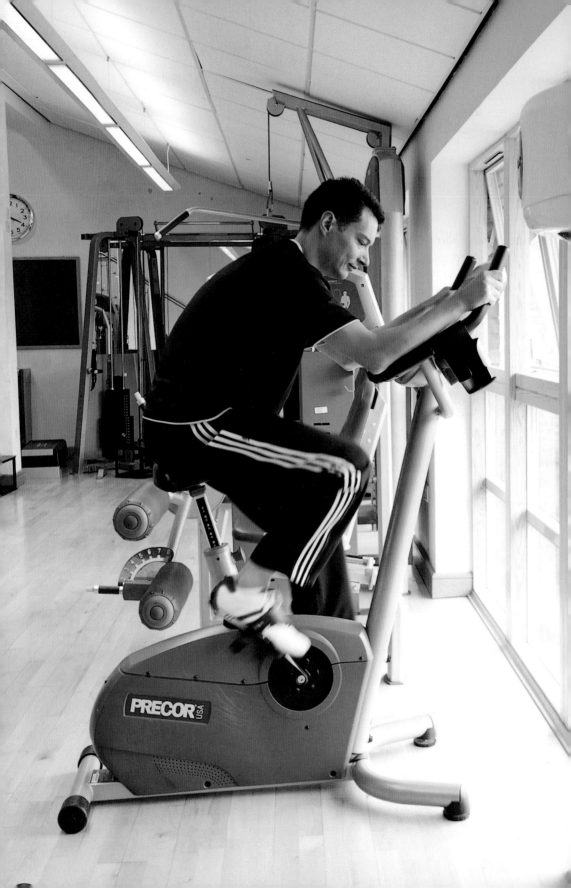

# 1    Introduction

*Anyone who takes part in sport will train using a range of sport-specific and non sport-specific drills. If your training is focused on just one particular form of exercise then it may be that in some respects you are very fit; however, there may be other aspects of your fitness that require work. For example, someone who does a lot of running or cycling might have good stamina, but their flexibility or upper body strength may be quite weak. Similarly, someone who may be very flexible might not be able to do any press-ups, or be able to coordinate complicated movement sequences.*

*This book introduces the different components of fitness. Its aim is to enable anyone involved in sports training to identify and develop areas which might need further work. If you are not aware of the various types of fitness training that you could be doing, you may have inadvertently missed out certain types of training. As a result, your overall fitness levels might not be what you were aiming for through your efforts.*

*Total Fitness looks at eleven different components of fitness in turn and considers what exercises can be done to improve the various aspects. These components are outlined in the table overleaf.*

*By knowing that there are a number of different ways in which you can train, you should be able to take more effective decisions about how to improve your fitness.*

---

### The Components of Fitness

The eleven components of fitness:

- **strength**            – exerting force

- **strength endurance**    – withstanding fatigue

- **power**            – generating large amounts of force in short periods of time

- **plyometrics**       – increasing power using the stretch-shortening cycle

- **stamina**          – sustaining low level aerobic work for a long period of time

- **speed**            – moving the whole body or limbs quickly

- **agility**           – changing direction rapidly

- **coordination**      – moving body parts in a specific sequence

- **posture**          – maintaining efficient body alignment

- **flexibility**        – utilizing the full range of movement around a joint

- **balance**          – maintaining a state of equilibrium

---

# HOW TO USE THIS BOOK

### Chapter 2 – Training Tips

This chapter takes a look at some common training tips, such as warming up, cooling down and the kind of equipment that could be used during training. It also describes key safety considerations to be aware of when taking up any form of exercise or training regime.

### Chapter 3 – Understanding your Body

This chapter gives a brief introduction to human anatomy in the context of movement and exercise. It is intended to be a useful reference guide for identification of the muscles being used and the parts of the body that the various exercises impact upon. Having a basic understanding of how the muscular and skeletal system work together to create movement can be useful background knowledge for any person involved in fitness training.

### Chapters 4 to 12 – The Fitness Exercise Chapters

These chapters look at each of the fitness components in turn and give some brief information about them, the benefits of training for each one and also a range of exercises that could be used to develop each particular component. The chapters are as follows:

The exercises in this book tend to focus on those that do not require any special equipment. If any equipment is required, this will be mentioned within the exercise description. The exercises are suitable for a range of ability levels, so it is hoped that everyone will be able to adapt the exercises to match their developmental needs.

**Chapter 13 – Quick Reference Guides**
This chapter is a visual summary of the exercises described in this book. It can be used to provide a quick reference guide for support either during training, or as a reminder of what type of exercises can be useful for developing a particular fitness area. Over time, you may want to change your regular training programme, so these tables can be used to identify the types of exercises that could be incorporated into your programme. It should also help to highlight if there are particular areas of training that are being missed in your current fitness programme.

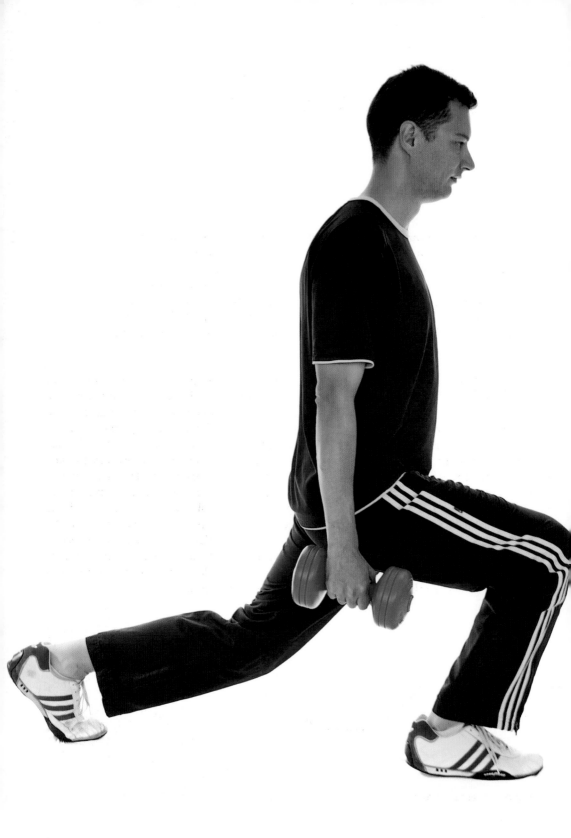

# 2   Training Tips

*Some general tips regarding training and safety that should be taken into account whilst using the exercises in the book are given in this chapter, including:*

- *reviewing your training*
- *keeping a training diary*
- *establishing your training objectives*

- *using a step-by-step approach*
- *measuring your progress*
- *training safely*
- *finding a suitable training environment*
- *using appropriate training equipment*
- *warming up as part of your workout*
- *cooling down as part of your workout.*

## REVIEWING YOUR TRAINING

There are a number of ways to approach your fitness training. Perhaps you are already aware of which areas of fitness you wish to develop, in which case you are likely to be tempted to go directly to those chapters. If you are currently heavily involved in sports, you will probably already have a good idea of what type of training is likely to be most beneficial to improving your performance, or, indeed, is most likely to help reduce the risk of injury. On the other hand, you may not be sure what your fitness level is, or where you should start, in which case you should steadily work through the exercises in this book, making a note of your progress in order to establish what aspects of your training would most benefit from immediate attention. You could use the table shown overleaf to make notes on each exercise as you do it. This should assist you in deciding where to focus your training efforts. Use the table as a template and work on a photocopy each time you do an exercise. In this way, you will be able to keep track of how you improve over time.

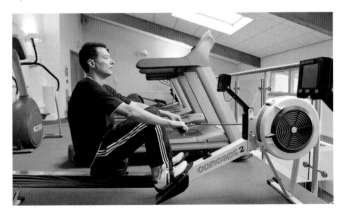

Rowing as a warm-up exercise.

| EXERCISE | YOUR NOTES | EXERCISE | YOUR NOTES |
|---|---|---|---|

**Strength, strength endurance and power training**
- partial press-up
- press-up
- back extension
- back extension with Swiss Ball
- triceps kick back
- triceps push-up
- crunch
- reverse crunch
- side crunch
- opposites crunch
- dumb-bell shrug
- dumb-bell press
- dumb-bell flye
- dumb-bell curl
- lateral raise
- bent-over lateral raise
- forward lunge
- reverse lunge
- squat

**Plyometric training**
- small jumps
- medium jumps
- step jumps
- knee tucks
- jump squats
- jumping for distance
- hopping for distance
- bounding for distance
- vertical press-ups with a hand clap
- horizontal press-ups with a hand clap

**Stamina training**
- skipping
- jogging
- swimming
- cycling
- rowing
- stair climbing
- star jump and press-up combination

**Speed training**
- skipping with alternating feet
- jumping in and out
- jumping side to side
- running
- downhill running

- uphill running
- running up steps
- acceleration exercises

**Agility training**
- 90-degree turn
- 180-degree turn
- 270-degree turn
- stepping forward with the leading leg and changing direction
- pulling back foot and stepping backward
- pulling back foot and stepping backward with change of direction
- moving backward and forward with a split step
- chassé and side step

**Coordination training**
- catching using one ball
- catching using two balls
- shuttlecock tapping
- skipping
- arms rotation
- punching
- upper-level block
- mid-level block
- low-level block
- same side split jump
- opposite sides split jump
- step and punch
- step and block
- step and opposite punch
- step and opposite block

**Posture training**
- looking forward
- standing with arms and legs out
- sitting with the legs in front
- sitting kneeling
- sitting cross-legged
- bridging
- donkey
- dog
- donkey with lifted arm
- walking

*(continued...)*

| EXERCISE | YOUR NOTES | EXERCISE | YOUR NOTES |
|---|---|---|---|
| **Flexibility training** | | **Balance training** | |
| • arm lifts in front | | • balls of the feet stand | |
| • arm lifts to the side | | • tandem feet stand | |
| • triceps stretch | | | |
| | | | |
| • calves stretch | | • heel stand | |
| • standing hip adductors stretch | | • one-legged stand | |
| • hamstring stretch | | • one-legged stand on ball of the foot | |
| • standing quadriceps stretch | | • holding one leg behind | |
| • sitting hip adductors stretch | | • holding one leg in front | |
| • lying quadriceps stretch | | • holding one leg to the side | |
| • gluteals stretch | | • walking on the balls of the feet | |
| • leaning backward | | • walking heel to toe | |
| • waist twist | | • walking heel to toe backward | |
| | | • walking on the heels | |
| | | • cross walking | |
| | | • jump | |
| | | • hop | |

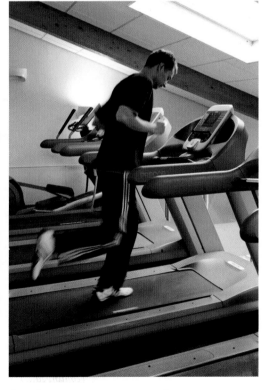

Jogging as a warm-up exercise.

## KEEPING A TRAINING DIARY

Keeping an activity and nutrition diary will encourage you to keep up with your training and also make you more aware of how you are coping with your training programme. If you have trouble keeping to the programme that you set yourself, you will need to revisit it and come up with something more achievable. A regular review and training diary together should enable you to vary your training programme as and when appropriate.

## ESTABLISHING YOUR TRAINING OBJECTIVES

When you are thinking about what type of training to do, you should have a clear idea in your mind about what you wish to achieve from any training programme. In this way, you can check that you are achieving what you intended and, if not, can reconsider your plan to see where it could

13

be improved. Complete the table below by deciding how much priority you place on a particular reason for exercising. The contents of the table should help you to think about why you wish to improve your fitness in the first place.

---

**Prioritizing the Reasons for Training**

| REASON | PRIORITY |
| --- | --- |

- To improve my fitness.
- To take up a new sport or activity.
- To improve in a sport or activity in which I am already taking part.
- To improve my appearance.
- To get back to a previous fitness level.
- To develop physically in a more holistic way.
- To include training which my sport or activity does not address.
- To rehabilitate after an injury.
- To meet new people.
- To have fun.

---

## USING A STEP-BY-STEP APPROACH

Most of the exercises shown in this book are presented using a step-by-step approach. By using this method you should be able to establish which steps you can complete in any given exercise. This should allow you to track your progress as you achieve more of the steps. If you later take a break in your training, you will be able to check if there is any reduction in your fitness levels by looking at your training notes.

## MEASURING YOUR PROGRESS

Training for fitness can be a slow and gradual process, so you will need to persevere with regular training to see the benefits. Do not expect just one or two sessions to show marked progress. It may take four to five sessions before you begin to feel any improvement. Fitness training is not a race. You must allow your body the time it needs

---

**Training Tips**

The following are some tips to help you during training:

- Where an exercise is shown using one side of the body, ensure that you train equally on both sides.

- If you are unable to work through all the steps of a particular exercise, just go as far as you are able. After repeated practice it should be possible to go further.

- None of the exercises should cause you pain or undue stress.

- You should not attempt any exercises that you are uncomfortable with.

---

to develop. It is best to train regularly. Two to three times a week should certainly be enough to start showing some benefits. Breaks in training will inevitably result in you feeling less fit. With time, training should become something that merges more and more into your everyday life, affecting how you move and feel each day.

To establish your ability level with respect to each exercise, you can work your way through Chapters 4 to 12 and, as well as using the training review and keeping a training diary, put a date against the exercises you can already perform. Use the anatomical diagrams in Chapter 3 in order to identify the muscles groups that you need to work on. Then, given time and through your practice, you can monitor your progress by putting dates against the more advanced steps as you achieve them. Through this process you will be able to track your progress and use this book to motivate you in your training.

## TRAINING SAFELY

As a prerequisite to joining a fitness class, most instructors are likely to request that you to complete a health check form. Alternatively, they may just ask you about any injuries or limitations they need to be aware of. Ensure that you let an instructor know of any relevant information so that they can carry out appropriate supervision of your training. Fitness instructors are generally not qualified to give medical advice, so participants should seek appropriate professional medical advice before taking part in any activity. Equally, if you are taking up a sport or activity as a method of rehabilitating after an injury or other trauma, you should consult an appropriate medical professional about what types of exercises and activities may be appropriate.

> **Important!**
>
> This book is intended to complement training done under the supervision of a trained instructor and is no substitute for a teacher.

## FINDING A SUITABLE TRAINING ENVIRONMENT

When selecting an area in which to train, you must ensure that it is suitable for the activity you are planning. There should be sufficient space in which to perform the exercise and it should be clear of any hazards. For example, you may want to move furniture or other objects out of the way. Also, check the floor

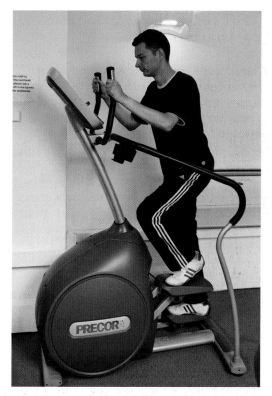

Using a step machine as a warm-up exercise.

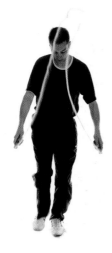

Skipping as a warm-up exercise.

would be useful for particular exercises is described in the appropriate chapter with the appropriate exercise. However, there are some key pieces of equipment that will make your training more comfortable and safe. It is essential to wear appropriate training clothes. These normally consist of T-shirts and jogging bottoms or shorts. Good shoes are also essential, if you are planning to do any kind of impact training, like running and jogging, or a high-impact exercise like jumping.

Although not essential for training, it can be useful to have a stopwatch, particularly for exercises aimed at improving speed, or in which you perform a particular exercise or sequence. A stopwatch can be used to monitor progress by counting how many repetitions you can complete within a fixed amount of time. This will allow you to see if you can beat your personal best each time you practise.

Where safety equipment is available, it is advised that you use it. For example, if you plan to cycle, wear a cycle helmet and appropriate clothing. If you have any injuries or require any kind of support, you should only train using the appropriate safety equipment.

for any holes or objects that are likely to cause trouble. The floor should not be slippery and should ideally be sprung so that you are supported during exercise. Training halls with mirrors can be useful, as they enable you to check your alignment and may also motivate you to keep going with your exercises.

It is best to train in a warm environment; if your training environment is really cold, an extended warm-up is recommended. Fitness training can be quite repetitive, so some people find it easier to practise while listening to music. Music with a regular beat may encourage you to keep up with a certain pace of exercise. If you do use music, however, ensure that it does not compromise your safety, for example if you are jogging or cycling outdoors.

## USING APPROPRIATE TRAINING EQUIPMENT

The emphasis in this book is on exercises that do not require any special equipment. However, there are some exercises that do require equipment, or could be made more challenging through its use. Equipment that

## WARMING UP AS PART OF YOUR WORKOUT

There are two main reasons for doing a warm-up. The first is to reduce the risk of injury and the second is to improve your performance during the activity. Blood flow to the muscles is increased during a warm-up, the joints become lubricated and the heart rate increases. Warming up should also lead to greater performance from your muscles, by extending the amount of time before fatigues sets in. A warm-up should consist of around ten minutes of continuous aerobic activity, such as jogging or using a step machine. The exercises shown here could be used as warm-up exercises. They are described in detail later in this book.

They should raise your body temperature and make you sweat a little. This should be followed by exercises that take the joints through the range of motion. In particular, those joints should be warmed-up that will later be involved in the activity.

## COOLING DOWN AS PART OF YOUR WORKOUT

A cool-down period after training is often recommended. The aim of this is to reduce the heart rate and help to remove fluid build-up from around the muscles. Static stretching is often recommended for this part of the workout. The exercises shown here could be used as cool-down exercises. They are described in detail later in this book.

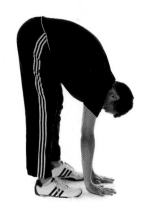

Hamstring stretch as a cool-down exercise.

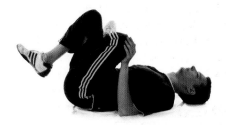

Gluteals stretch as a cool-down exercise.

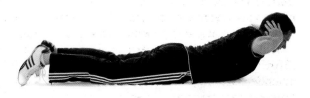

Back extension as a cool-down exercise.

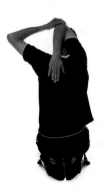

Triceps stretch as a cool-down exercise.

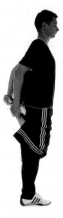

Quadriceps stretch as a cool-down exercise.

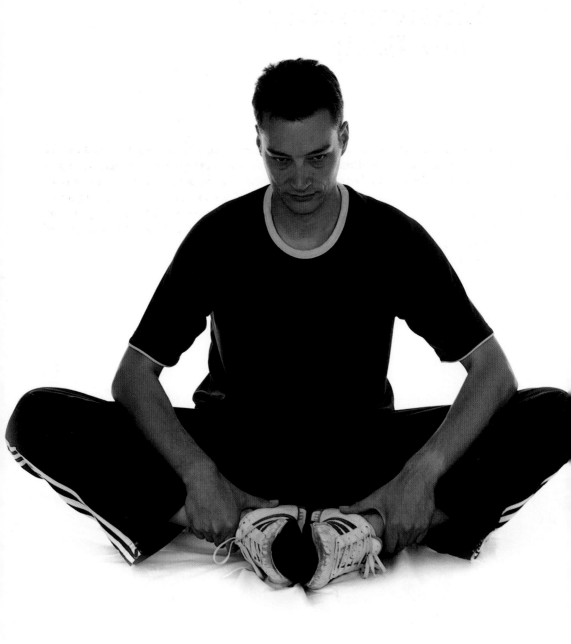

# 3   Understanding Your Body

*It can be useful for anyone taking part in sports and fitness activities to have a basic understanding of how the body moves. This chapter looks at the following areas:*
* *the skeletal system*
* *movement terminology*
* *the different types of joints*
* *the muscular system.*

*While performing any exercise, it can be beneficial to think about how you are using your joints and also which muscles are taking part in the motion. You should use the diagrams in this chapter as quick reference guides, so that you can inform any queries you may have about your training and development.*

## THE SKELETAL SYSTEM

All of the bones in the body form the skeleton. They provide the structures that the muscles connect to and act on. Muscles can contract or extend, and it is this action that creates the movement around the joints of the body. As well as enabling motion, the function of the skeleton is also to protect the organs of the body.

The skeleton can be considered in two parts (see illustration on page 21). Firstly, the axial skeleton, which supports the head, neck and trunk. This consists of the skull, the vertebral column, the ribs and the sternum. Secondly, the appendicular skeleton, which supports the appendages, or limbs, and attaches them to the rest of the body. This consists of the shoulder girdle, the upper limbs, the pelvic girdle and the lower limbs. The shoulder girdle comprises the clavicle, the scapula and the humerus. The pelvic girdle comprises the innominate bones, the sacrum, the femur, the coccyx and the symphysis pubis. The wrist comprises eight carpal bones and the hand comprises five metacarpal bones. The fingers are composed of fourteen phalanges in each hand, two in the thumb and three in each of the fingers. The ankle and the foot comprise seven tarsals and five metatarsals. The toes are composed of fourteen phalanges in each foot, two in the big toe and three in each of the other toes.

## MOVEMENT TERMINOLOGY

Fitness professionals often use specific terminology to describe the movement of the body. Knowing this terminology can be useful in terms of understanding what a particular exercise does or why it is called a particular name, especially if the name includes the definition of the movement. The main types of motion are shown in the diagrams on pages 22 and 23.

## THE DIFFERENT TYPES OF JOINTS

The skeleton provides the joints in the body on which the muscles can act to create movement. The main joint types involved in movement are shown in the diagram on page 24.

## THE MUSCULAR SYSTEM

It is the muscles that are attached to the skeleton that enable movement, therefore understanding the muscular system is fundamental to understanding the effect of exercise on the body. During challenging exercise, the muscles use a lot of the oxygen and blood supply of the body, so the effect of exercise on the muscles can impact on other parts of the body.

The nervous system sends the muscles a signal and it is this that actions the muscles to contract to deliver the movement. The muscle fibres are bound together into bundles and it is these that attach to the bones through the tendons. These form the musculo-tendinous units. Tendons are strong sheets of connective tissues like ligaments. Tendons attach muscle to bone and ligaments attach bone to bone. Exercise, particularly strength training, can increase the effectiveness of the muscle attachment to the bone through the tendons. When the muscle contracts, it shortens and becomes thicker in the centre. On extension, the muscle lengthens out again, becoming thinner in the centre. This is enabled by the elastic nature of the muscular tissue.

Muscles tend to work in pairs, so that as one muscle group contracts, another will be extending. This is often called the contracting and relaxing of muscles respectively. When you bend your knee, it is the muscles in the back of the leg that contract and the muscles in the front of the leg that

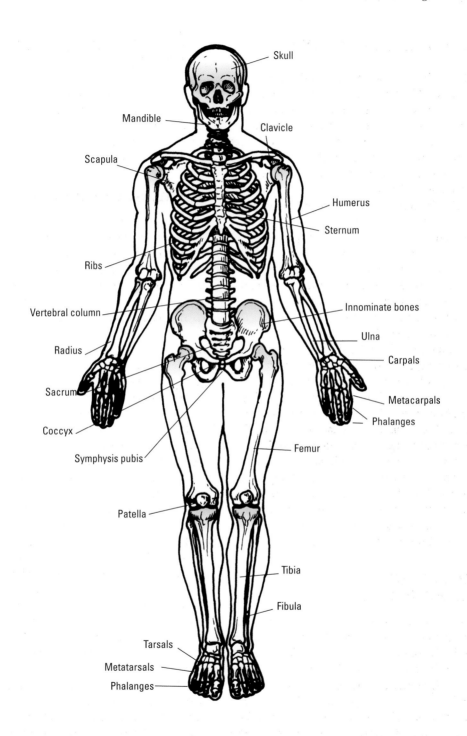

The skeletal system.

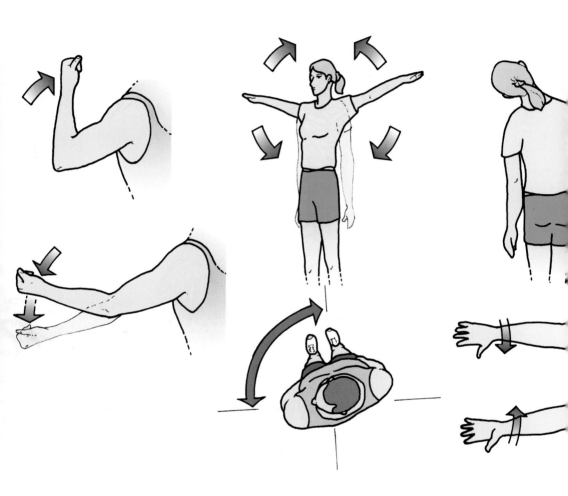

Types of movement 1.

relax. In order to produce smooth movement and reduce the risk of injury, it is important that the degree of muscle relaxation and contraction within the action is equal. Stretching and training in yoga and pilates can serve to highlight any imbalances in action. Even when the body is relaxed, the muscles will tend to hold a certain degree of contraction. This is known as muscle tone and it helps the body to maintain posture. It is possible to relax these muscles further using conscious effort.

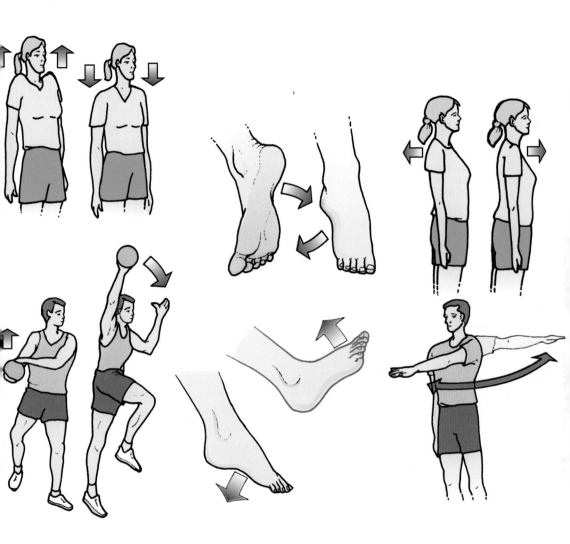

Types of movement 2.

The blood supplies the muscles with oxygen and nutrients that are required for movement. The blood is also responsible for taking away any waste products that build up during exercise, such as lactic acid and urea. Muscle performance can be affected by the following factors:

• the amount of energy available
• the strength of the signal from the nervous system
• the length of time the muscle has been

23

# Joint Types

## Slightly moveable joint

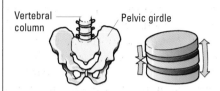

Also known as a cartilaginous joint. It moves by the compression of the cartilage between the bones, for example in the vertebral column.

## Ball and socket joint

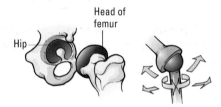

The most moveable of all joints. Allows flexion, extension, adduction, abduction, rotation and circumduction, for example, in the shoulder and hip joints.

## Hinge joint

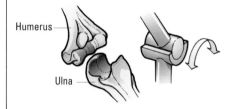

Allows movement in one direction or plane only. Movements are flexion and extension in, for example, the elbow, the knee, the ankle, the joints between the phalanges of the fingers and the toes.

## Gliding joint

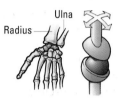

Allows bones to glide over each other, for example between the tarsals and between the carpals.

## Pivot joint

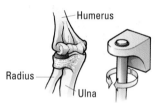

Allows movement around one axis only. This is a rotary movement, for example, in the radius and the ulna joint.

## Saddle joint

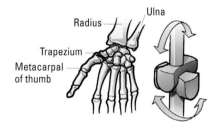

Allows movement around two axes, allowing flexion, extension, adduction, abduction, circumduction, for example in the wrist.

contracting
• sufficient oxygen and nutrients made available from the blood supply
• the temperature of the muscle (warmth increases the response)
• the presence of waste products such as lactic acid and urea.

The muscular system diagrams on pages 26 and 27 can be a useful guide to recognizing which of the major muscle groups you will be working in the various exercises that you perform, particularly when looking at the strength, flexibility, posture and balance training chapters. This should help you to understand your training programme more thoroughly and to suggest additions if you feel there are certain areas that are being neglected. Knowing the right terminology should also make it easier for you to communicate with fitness professionals.

Some of the muscle groups have commonly used names. These include the:

• quadriceps (full name quadriceps femoris): consists of the rectus femoris, the vastus lateralis, the vastus medialis and the vastus intermedius; the vastus intermedius is located between the vastus lateralis and the vastus medialis and is below the rectus femoris
• hamstrings: consists of the biceps femoris, the semi-tendinous and the semi-membranosus
• hip adductors: consists of the adductor brevis, the adductor longus and the adductor magnus; all three of these originate on the pubis and the adductor brevis is situated behind the adductor longus.

Further information on the muscular system can be found in Norris (2001), Lamb (1984) and Bean (2001).

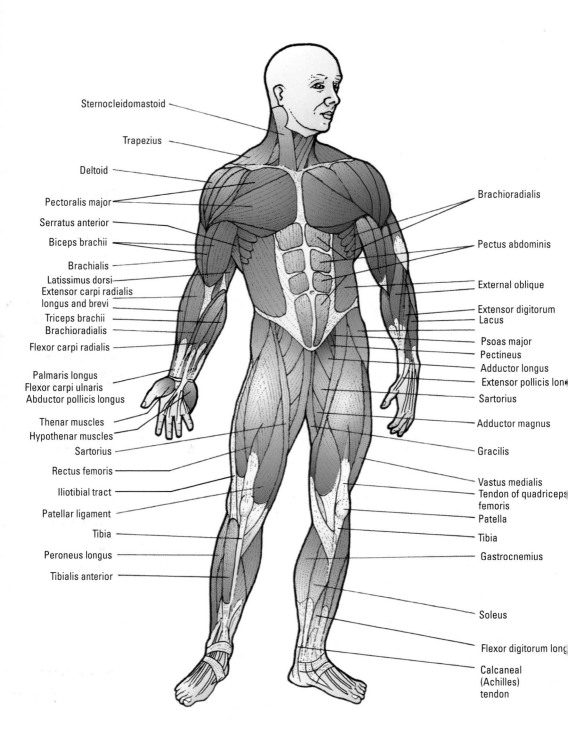

Sternocleidomastoid

Trapezius

Deltoid

Pectoralis major

Serratus anterior

Biceps brachii

Brachialis

Latissimus dorsi
Extensor carpi radialis
longus and brevi

Triceps brachii
Brachioradialis

Flexor carpi radialis

Palmaris longus
Flexor carpi ulnaris
Abductor pollicis longus

Thenar muscles
Hypothenar muscles

Sartorius

Rectus femoris

Iliotibial tract

Patellar ligament

Tibia

Peroneus longus

Tibialis anterior

Brachioradialis

Pectus abdominis

External oblique

Extensor digitorum
Lacus

Psoas major
Pectineus
Adductor longus
Extensor pollicis lon

Sartorius

Adductor magnus

Gracilis

Vastus medialis
Tendon of quadriceps
femoris
Patella

Tibia

Gastrocnemius

Soleus

Flexor digitorum long

Calcaneal
(Achilles)
tendon

The muscles at the front of the body.

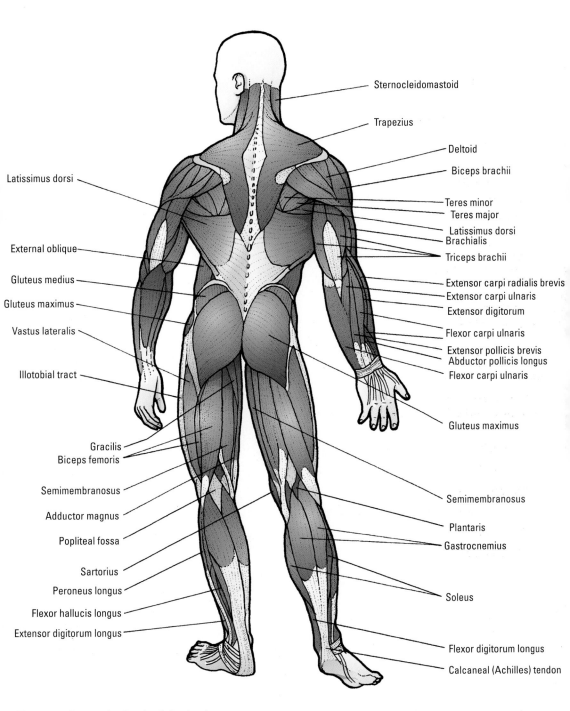

Sternocleidomastoid

Trapezius

Deltoid

Biceps brachii

Teres minor
Teres major

Latissimus dorsi
Brachialis

Triceps brachii

Extensor carpi radialis brevis
Extensor carpi ulnaris

Extensor digitorum

Flexor carpi ulnaris

Extensor pollicis brevis
Abductor pollicis longus

Flexor carpi ulnaris

Gluteus maximus

Latissimus dorsi

External oblique

Gluteus medius

Gluteus maximus

Vastus lateralis

Illotobial tract

Gracilis
Biceps femoris

Semimembranosus

Adductor magnus

Popliteal fossa

Sartorius

Peroneus longus

Flexor hallucis longus

Extensor digitorum longus

Semimembranosus

Plantaris

Gastrocnemius

Soleus

Flexor digitorum longus

Calcaneal (Achilles) tendon

The muscles at the back of the body.

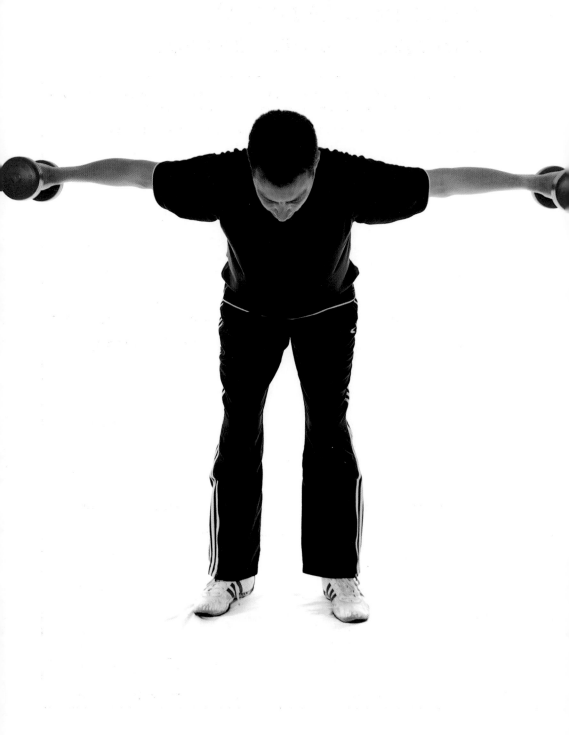

# 4 Strength, Strength Endurance and Power

*Strength: the capacity to exert force. Strength endurance: the capacity of the muscles to withstand fatigue. Power: the capacity to generate large amounts of force in short periods of time.*

**Strength, Strength Endurance and Power Training Exercises Summary**

Ground exercises:

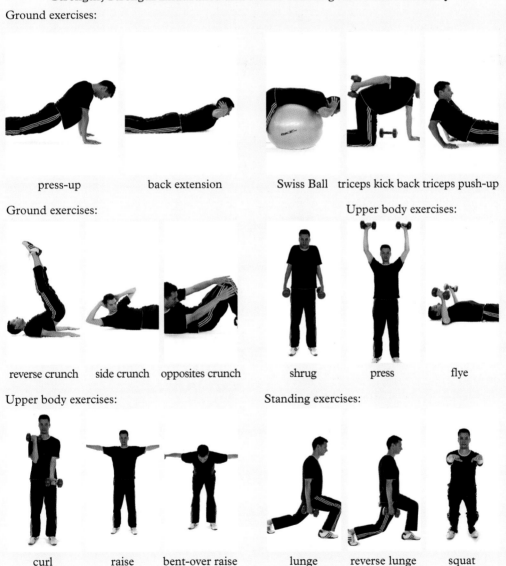

| press-up | back extension | Swiss Ball | triceps kick back | triceps push-up |

Ground exercises:                    Upper body exercises:

| reverse crunch | side crunch | opposites crunch | shrug | press | flye |

Upper body exercises:                Standing exercises:

| curl | raise | bent-over raise | lunge | reverse lunge | squat |

# ABOUT STRENGTH, STRENGTH ENDURANCE AND POWER

## Strength

Strength training is about building the strength, endurance and size of the muscles. Exercise examples include how much you can lift and how hard you can push. These exercises normally take the form of resistance training, which can be either training against gravity, using only your own partial or full body weight, or using weights. Weights can take the form of free weights, such as dumb-bells and sandbags, or fixed weights, such as those used in gym equipment. The objective is gradually to increase the resistance applied over time.

## Strength Endurance

Strength endurance is the capacity of muscles to withstand fatigue by demonstrating strength over a prolonged period of time. Sports that involve strength endurance are numerous in nature, from swimming to fighting. An example would be how long you could hold a position or a weight before muscle fatigue set in. This could include holding positions such as the forward lunge or dumb-bell press described later in this chapter.

## Power

Power is the combination of force and speed. Strength training can improve your power through improvement in the force part of the equation. In order to improve the speed component, rapid repetitions with lighter weights is a technique that is commonly used.

Plyometrics is also a type of power training and this is covered separately in Chapter 5. Untrained individuals can significantly improve their power through weight training. Once a plateau in your power is reached, however, it is time to consider more sport-specific power training. If you want to increase the strength of your punch, kick or some action, then you may want to include plyometric training in your programme.

## Why are Strength, Strength Endurance and Power Considered Together?

The exercises in this chapter are general strength training exercises. Such training can develop all three of the fitness components of strength, strength endurance and power. The amount of weight that you use, the number of repetitions and the speed of the action will determine which component you will be developing more. This means that you can use the same exercises, as presented in this chapter, to focus on any of these three components by varying the weight, repetitions and speed of the action. You can use the following guidelines to help you:

- developing strength: use heavier weights and lower repetitions
- developing strength endurance: use lighter weights and increase the number of repetitions
- developing power: use even lighter weights, further increase the repetitions and make the action faster.

# BENEFITS OF TRAINING FOR STRENGTH, STRENGTH ENDURANCE AND POWER

According to Bean (2001), strength training is believed to result in the following improvements:

- raised metabolic rate and reduced body fat and blood pressure
- improved appearance, muscle tone and posture
- increased bone density
- increased muscle strength and mass
- increased tendon and ligament strength
- improved joint function
- decreased age-related muscle loss.

Strength training develops the muscles and this in turn increases the basal metabolic rate of the individual. For this reason, strength training is often part of a fat loss programme. Indeed, intense workouts will also have the effect of increasing the metabolic rate for several hours after training, which should reduce the amount of fat laid down from food eaten soon after training. Like any type of training, strength training can help you to feel good about yourself and more energetic. Strength training can help to improve performance in all sports.

## Combating Muscle Loss

Strength training can delay the effects of aging by reducing muscle loss due to age, which can result in older people being less frail. Strength training can reduce the risk of injury by making the muscles stronger and more able to cope with the demands put upon them. Cardiovascular training alone will not help to combat muscle loss and so strength training is normally recommended as part of most people's training programme. It can help you to stay in good shape and maintain a healthy posture. For this reason, it is essential to find a way to incorporate it into your lifestyle.

### Triggering Growth Hormones

Strength training is believed to be effective in releasing growth hormones to build cartilage, muscle and bone. Muscles will develop in response to the demands that are put on them. Bones then grow dependent on the stresses that the muscles exert on them. When training, the number of repetitions should be kept low and the amount of weight built up instead. This is in order to get the right type of activity to release the growth hormones. If you can do more than three to five repetitions you are working on the strength endurance range and power range of the exercise. This will tend to burn fat and increase muscular endurance, but won't trigger as much growth hormone to build muscle. This is why training is done with smaller repetitions and in sets of activity. This way, each set can maximize muscle growth.

# IMPROVING STRENGTH, STRENGTH ENDURANCE AND POWER

There are number of ways in which to carry out a strength training programme that can result in faster improvements. Initially, though, you would start by trying to increase the number of repetitions, the duration of exercise, the weight or resistance, or reducing the recovery periods between sets of repetitions. A guideline table for repetitions is given below. However, this should be adjusted to reflect your own ability level and should be varied as you develop. The more you train, you should have an improved sense of what number of repetitions and weights makes sense for your goals. Further information can be found in Bean (2001) and Roberts (2005).

| Varying the resistance and repetitions for focusing on strength, strength endurance or power | | |
|---|---|---|
| **Training objective** | **Resistance based on your ability** | **Repetitions** |
| Strength | 75–90% | 1–5 |
| Strength endurance | 50–75% | 5–20 |
| Power | < 50% | 20 + |

**Free Weights versus Fixed Weights**

Free weights are good for training because they make you balance, using stabilizing muscles, thus engaging a number of different muscles to achieve the movement. When using machines, you are more likely to isolate muscles and make them bigger while working less of your muscles overall, so for more well-rounded fitness training it can be better to use free weights.

## SAFETY CONSIDERATIONS

Strength training is a safe form of exercise when the movements are slow, controlled and carefully defined. However, as with any form of exercise, improper execution and the failure to take appropriate precautions can result in injury. When using any form of resistance, you will need to ensure that you work within your limitations and ability level. Any increase in the amount of resistance used should be gradually and carefully introduced.

## STRENGTH, STRENGTH ENDURANCE AND POWER EXERCISES

**Partial Press-Up**

This exercise is a simplified version of the normal press-up and is good for developing upper body strength. You should feel the work being done in the arms, chest and the back in particular. Unlike a regular press-up, this exercise reduces the weight that the body works against by bending at the knees. In this way, only partial body weight is used in the exercise, therefore making it a suitable starting point for anyone who has trouble doing a full press-up like that shown in the next exercise.

Start on the ground with your hands directly underneath the shoulders, with your lower legs raised off the ground. Next, lift up by pushing off from your hands in a controlled manner until your arms are straight. Lower yourself slowly, aiming to avoid any jerkiness in the movement. If you

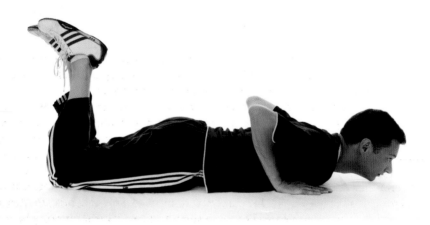

Step 1. Place your hands in line with your shoulders while lying on the ground, face down. Keep your knees together. Bend at your knees, so that your lower legs are raised. Ensure that your knees are in contact with the ground.

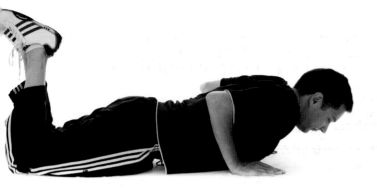

Step 2. Look towards the ground and begin to lift your weight upwards. Try to use a slow and controlled motion.

Step 3. Keep pushing your upper body upwards until your arms are straight. Keep your back straight. Your weight should then be on your palms and knees. Return into the position in Step 1. Again, ensure that you use a slow and controlled motion rather than dropping down. Repeat as required.

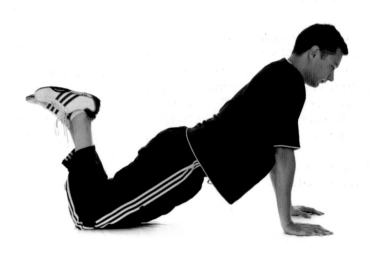

are new to this type of exercise, you may find it quite difficult. In which case, start off by attempting between five and ten repetitions, building up as you become stronger over time. The eventual aim is to be able to perform the full press-up.

**Press-Up**

This is the more advanced version of the previous exercise and is also useful for building upper body strength. You should feel the work being done in the arms, chest and the back in particular. The full body weight is supported on the palms and the balls of the feet in the end position. You will

need to focus on keeping the body straight as you lift yourself up and come down again in a controlled manner.

Start on the ground with your hands directly underneath the shoulders and the balls of your feet in contact with the ground. Next, lift up by pushing off from your hands until your arms are straight. Lower yourself slowly, aiming to avoid any jerkiness in the movement. If you are new to this type of exercise, start off by attempting between five and ten repetitions, building up as you become stronger over time. The eventual aim is to be able to perform the full press-up as effortlessly as possible.

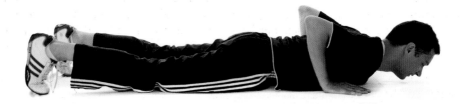

Step 1. Place your hands in line with your shoulders while lying on the ground, face down. The balls of your feet should be in contact with the ground. Keep your legs hip-width apart in this exercise.

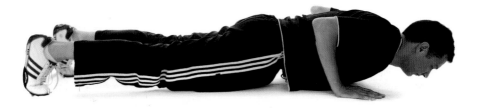

Step 2. Look towards the ground and begin to lift your weight upwards. Focus on keeping your back straight. Use a slow and controlled motion.

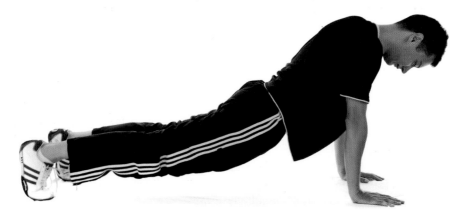

Step 3. Continue to push up until your arms are straight. Your weight should then be on your palms and the balls of your feet. Return to the position in Step 1. Use a slow and controlled motion rather than dropping down. Repeat as required.

## Back Extension

This exercise focuses on developing the muscles along the erector spinae, particularly in the lower back, and the gluteals. It focuses on extending the back outwards. These muscles are often used in stabilizing the body, so developing these muscles in particular should help you to reduce the risk of injury when performing everyday tasks.

Start in a position on the ground face down, resting your hands on your head lightly so that no undue stress is applied. Next, lift your upper body off the ground as far as you are comfortable, then relax down again. You should complete this exercise using a smooth and continuous motion. If you are new to this type of exercise, you may find you are not very flexible in the back, meaning that you will not be able to extend very far back or may find it uncomfortable. With practice, this should improve and you should gradually be able to achieve an improved back extension over time. This exercise should not be attempted without specific medical advice if you have any back problems.

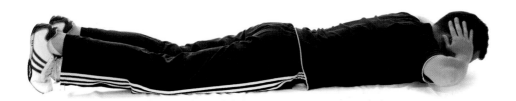

Step 1. Lie on the floor face down. Place your hands on either side of your head with your elbows pointing outwards. Do not put any pressure on your head through your hands. Ensure that the balls of your feet are in contact with the ground. Look towards the ground.

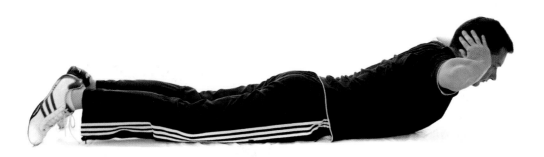

Step 2. Raise your upper body as far are you are able, hold for a moment and then relax. Keep the motion smooth and controlled throughout. Repeat as required.

**Back Extension with Swiss Ball**

This exercise also focuses on developing the muscles along the erector spinae, particularly in the lower back, and the gluteals. It focuses on extending the back outwards. You may find attempting the back extension using a Swiss Ball for support more comfortable than the previous exercise. These muscles are often used in stabilizing the body, so developing these muscles in particular should help to reduce the risk of injury when performing everyday tasks.

Start in a position with your weight resting on the Swiss Ball, resting your hands on your head lightly so that no undue stress is applied. Next, lift your upper body off the ball as far as you are comfortable and then relax down again. You should complete this exercise using a smooth and continuous motion. Ensure that you wear suitable footwear, so that you do not slip while leaning on the Swiss Ball. If this type of exercise is new to you, you may find that you are not very flexible in the back and therefore may not able to extend very far back or may find it uncomfortable. With practice, this should improve and you should gradually be able to achieve an improved back extension over time. This exercise should not be attempted without specific medical advice if you have any back problems.

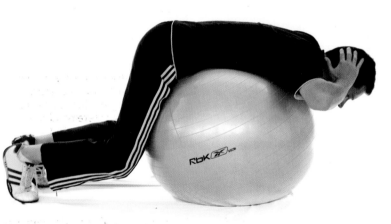

Step 1. Lie on the Swiss Ball face down. Place your hands on either side of your head with your elbows pointing outwards. Do not put any pressure on your head through your hands. Ensure that the balls of your feet are in contact with the ground and that you will not slip. Look towards the ground.

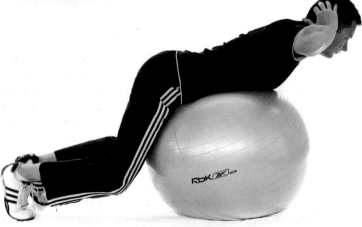

Step 2. Raise your upper body as far as you are able, hold for a moment and then relax. Aim to keep the motion smooth and controlled throughout. Repeat as required.

Step 1. Start in a position on your hands and knees. Hold a dumb-bell in one hand. Look at the ground. Ensure you are not holding any tension in your back, neck and shoulders. The elbow of your loaded arm should be in line with your body.

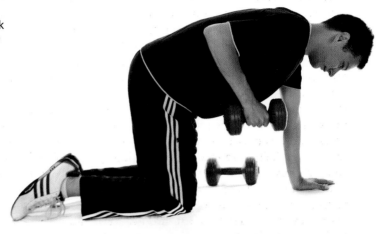

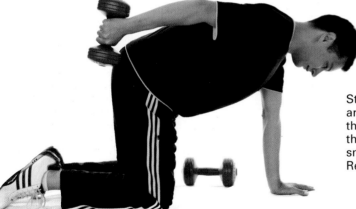

Step 2. Straighten the loaded arm behind you and return to the starting position. Ensure that the complete motion is smooth and controlled. Repeat as required.

## Triceps Kick Back

This exercise focuses on the development of the triceps. It is the first of a series of exercises in this chapter that uses dumb-bells.

Here, you start in a position on all fours, then hold a dumb-bell in one hand while keeping the elbow of that arm near your body. To perform the exercise, keep your upper arm stationary and straighten the arm by moving the forearm only. If too light a weight is used, you may be able to do too many repetitions of this exercise before muscle fatigues sets in. By increasing the weight until you are only able to do between three to five repetitions in one go, you will be working on improving muscle strength rather than power.

It is important to ensure that you use the correct weight for your ability level and your training goal. Once you find a particular weight too easy, you should consider attempting the exercise with a slightly heavier weight. Ensure that you keep your back and neck in a straight line and relaxed during the movement. Looking towards the ground will stop you from holding tension in your neck and shoulders.

**Triceps Push-Up**

This is another triceps exercise. However, this time you will be working against your own body weight. Here you start in a position on the ground with your palms supporting your weight underneath you. They should be near your hips. Lower your body as far as you can, then lift back up. It is important to carry out this exercise in a smooth and continuous manner. You may find this exercise far more difficult than the previous one, especially if you were only using light weights before.

Two versions of this exercise are shown. The first is performed on the ground and the second is performed using a support. You could start off by attempting ten repetitions of this exercise. Many students find this one particularly difficult because the triceps often get left out in training, so these muscles tend to be weaker than the other major muscles. With repeated practice, you should begin to find it easier to perform this exercise and this will indicate the speed at which your muscles are responding to the activity. You should feel the muscles working hard during the downward motion. Muscle fatigue can often set in quite quickly for untrained individuals during this exercise.

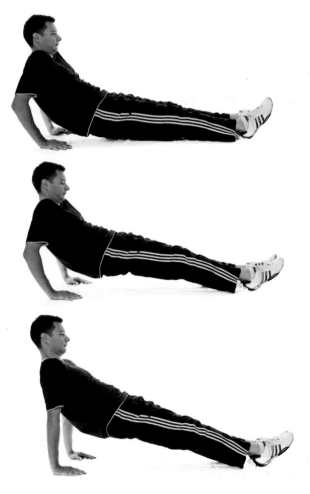

Step 1. Lie on the ground on your back. Place your palms on the ground just below your shoulders and near your hips.

Step 2. Start to raise the body off the ground, while trying to keep it straight.

Step 3. Hold for a moment, then relax down to the starting position in Step 1. Ensure that the complete motion is smooth and controlled. Repeat as required.

This exercise can also be attempted using a support, so that your starting point is higher off the ground. You may find it easier to use a raised support when first trying this exercise.

The raised support will also enable you to achieve a deeper dip as you come down. Again, you will feel the muscles working hard during the downward part of the exercise.

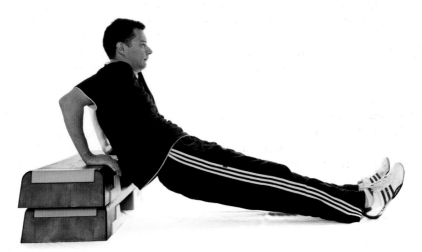

Step 1. Position yourself on the support ready for performing the triceps dip. Place your palms on the edge of the support just below your shoulders. Start to raise the body, while trying to keep it straight.

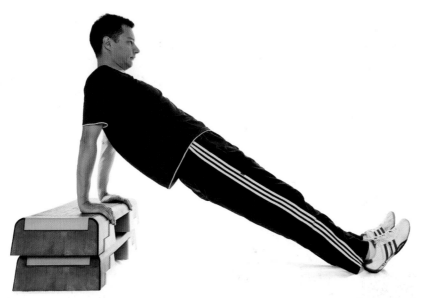

Step 2. Hold for a moment, then relax down to the starting position in Step 1. Ensure that the complete motion is smooth and controlled. Repeat as required.

## Crunch

There are a number of different ways in which you can work the muscles in the abdominal region. The exercise here is the first of four abdominal crunch exercises. It is the normal forward crunch, which predominantly works the upper abdominals. This normally needs to be combined with the reverse crunch so that the lower abdominals are also worked.

Start in a position lying on the ground with your knees bent. Rest your hands on the back of your head if that helps. However, you should not apply any pressure with your hands. This exercise is not like a sit-up, in that you are not trying to come all the way up. The aim is to curl your body up using predominantly your abdominal muscles in a slow and controlled manner, being careful

> **Engaging the Pelvic Floor Muscles**
>
> You can try this exercise holding your pelvic floor muscles in at the same time. To engage the pelvic floor, pull in the lower muscles as if trying to halt the flow of urine. It should feel like a zipping-up motion as these muscles are engaged. This technique can be added to many of the other exercises in this book.

not to put any undue stress on the neck or shoulders. Come up as far as your abdominals on their own allow you to. A good target to start with might be fifty repetitions. You could then try to build this up in sets of twenty-five.

Step 1. Lie on your back with your hands on your head and your feet flat on the ground.

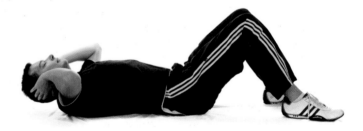

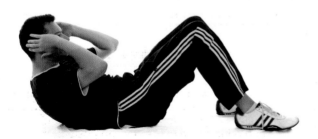

Step 2. Raise your head and shoulders off the ground by tightening your abdominals. Do not hold any tension in your neck. Hold for a moment, then relax down to the starting position in Step 1. Ensure that the complete motion is smooth and controlled. Repeat as required.

## Reverse Crunch

This exercise works the lower abdominals. It is often used in combination with the previous exercise in order to work the full range of the abdominals. In this exercise, you start off lying on the ground on your back with your legs pointing to the ceiling. From here, you should lift up your lower body using mostly the muscles in your abdominals.

Students often find this exercise far more difficult than the straightforward crunch. This is probably because the lower abdominals are more likely to be neglected during training, so may be much weaker than the upper abdominals. You should perform this exercise in a slow and controlled manner, being careful not to put any undue stress on your neck or shoulders. Come up as far as your abdominals on their own allow you to.

Try not to throw yourself while doing this exercise. A good target to start with might be twenty-five repetitions, building up in sets of five. You could consider engaging your pelvic floor muscles while doing this exercise. This exercise should not be attempted without medical advice if you have any back problems.

## Side Crunch

This is another form of the crunch type exercise. It works the obliques and the abdominal muscles. The exercise starts with you lying on your side. From here, you should use the muscles in the side of your body to enable you to perform the side crunch. Generally speaking, this exercise is easier than the previous two, the crunch and the reverse crunch. Again, you should focus on not holding any tension in your neck or shoulders and should make the movement in a slow and controlled fashion.

A good target to start with might be fifty repetitions on each side, building up in sets of twenty-five. Remember to complete this exercise equally on both sides. You could consider engaging the pelvic floor muscles while performing this exercise.

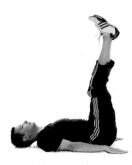

Step 1. Lie on your back with your hands by your side, with your legs raised straight and pointing to the ceiling.

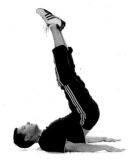

Step 2. Tighten your abdominals to enable you to lift your legs and hips off the ground. Keep your legs at ninety degrees to your body. Hold for a moment, then relax down to the starting position in Step 1. Ensure that the complete motion is smooth and controlled. Repeat as required.

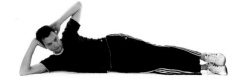

Step 1. Lie on the floor on your side with your hand supporting your head.

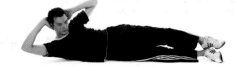

Step 2. Lift your raised shoulder further off the ground while tightening the muscles in the side of your body. Hold for a moment, then relax down to the starting position in Step 1. Ensure that the complete motion is smooth and controlled. Repeat as required.

## Opposites Crunch

This is another exercise that works the obliques and the abdominal muscles. You start off in a similar starting position to that in the crunch. However, this time your hands can rest on your legs. When you lift up, aim over to one side and then the other the next time you lift up. It is likely to be more tiring than a regular crunch. Again, you should focus on not holding any tension in your neck or shoulders and should make the movement in a slow and controlled fashion.

A good target to start with might be twenty-five repetitions on each side, building up in sets of twenty-five. Remember to complete this exercise equally on both sides. You could consider engaging the pelvic floor muscles while performing this exercise.

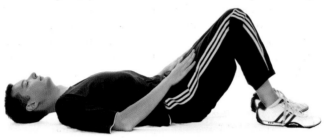

Step 1. Lie on your back with your hands resting on your legs and your feet flat on the ground. Your knees should be comfortably bent.

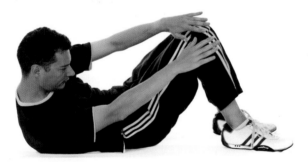

Step 2. Raise you head and shoulders off the ground and lift up, aiming towards one side. Do not hold any tension in your neck. Hold for a moment and then relax down to the starting position in Step 1.

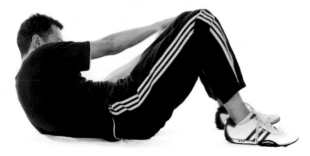

Step 3. Repeat the same motion on the other side of the body. Continue to repeat as required.

## Dumb-bell Shrug

This exercise develops the trapezius and other muscles around the shoulders. It is a simple exercise suitable for starting with, but care should be taken not to overload the muscles by using weights that are too heavy. Here this exercise is shown with dumb-bells, but you could try it with barbells instead. In which case, the barbell would be held in front of you. You should perform this exercise by starting off with the dumb-bells by your side, slowly lifting your shoulders then slowly dropping them as far as they will go. Your arms should remain by your sides throughout the exercise.

## Dumb-bell Press

This exercise develops the muscles in the chest. It is a medium-level exercise. Do not overload the muscles by using weights that are too heavy. Here this exercise is shown with dumb-bells, but you could try it with barbells instead, holding them in front of you then raising them above your head. You should perform this exercise by starting off with the dumb-bells by your shoulders and then slowly lifting the weights until your arms are straight. You should then return to your starting position using a slow and controlled motion.

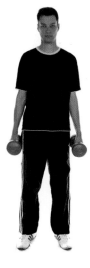

Step 1. Stand with your feet hip-width apart, holding a dumb-bell in each hand.

Step 1. Stand with your feet hip-width apart holding a dumb-bell in each hand at head level, just above your shoulders.

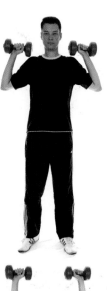

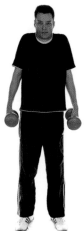

Step 2. Raise your shoulders, hold for a moment, then relax down again. Repeat as required.

Step 2. Raise the dumb-bells above your head, hold for a moment, then relax down again. Use a slow and controlled motion throughout. Repeat as required.

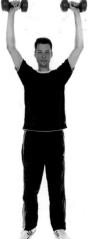

## Dumb-bell Flye

This exercise also develops the muscles in the chest. It is another medium-level exercise. Do not overload the muscles by using weights that are too heavy. You should perform this exercise by starting off with the dumb-bells lifted above you while lying on the ground. Move the dumb-bells in an arc motion (this is the meaning of 'flye'), then return to your starting position using a slow and controlled motion. Do not let the elbows go below your shoulder line on the downward motion.

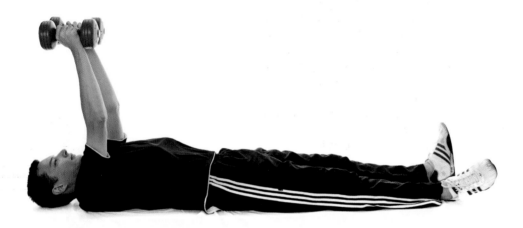

Step 1. Lie on your back on the ground. Hold the dumb-bells in each hand directly above you. There should be a slight bend in the elbows.

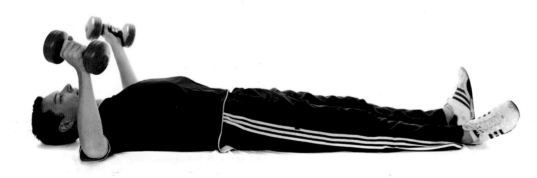

Step 2. Lower the dumb-bells to your side, using an arc motion, until just above the point at which your arms are in line with your shoulder. The elbows should be bent. Do not hold in this position. Continue through back to the position in Step 1. Use a slow and controlled motion throughout. Repeat as required.

## Dumb-bell Curl

This exercise develops the muscles around and including the biceps. It is a simple exercise suitable for starting with, but take care not to overload the muscles by using weights that are too heavy. Perform this exercise by starting off with holding the dumb-bells in front of you. You should then curl the dumb-bells in towards your body alternately using a slow and controlled motion. Do not be tempted to swing the dumb-bells, or to perform this exercise too quickly. The upper arms should remain stationary throughout the exercise, such that only the forearms are moving. You should also aim to straighten the arm fully in the downward motion, so that the maximum range of your muscles is engaged.

Step 1. Stand with your feet hip-width apart holding a dumb-bell in each hand in front of your body.

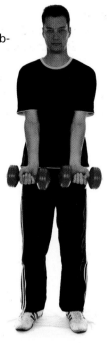

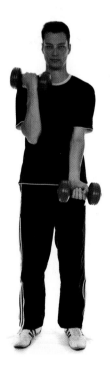

Step 2. Curl one dumb-bell up using only your forearm. At the top of the motion, your palm should face towards you.

Step 3. Uncurl that arm, then curl up the arm on other side. Remember that the arm going down should be completely straight at the bottom of the motion. Use a slow and controlled motion throughout. Repeat as required.

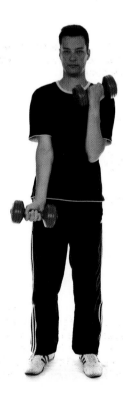

45

## Lateral Raise

This exercise develops the muscles around the upper body and shoulders. It is an exercise that looks simple, yet can be quite demanding. Take care not to overload the muscles by using weights that are too heavy. Perform this exercise by starting off with holding the dumb-bells by your sides. Your arms should be almost straight. Lift your arms out to your sides, keeping the elbows only slightly bent throughout the motion. Do not be tempted to swing the dumb-bells, or to perform this exercise too quickly. The rest of your body should remain stationary throughout the exercise. Aim to lift the weights so that they are in line with your shoulders at the top of the motion. The exercise should be performed with the feeling that your elbows are leading the movement rather than your hands.

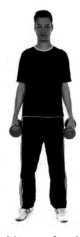 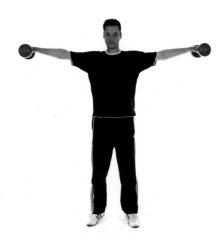

Step 1. Stand with your feet hip-width apart holding a dumb-bell in each hand by your side. Your arms should be slightly bent.

Step 2. Raise your arms to your sides until they are in line with your shoulders, hold for a moment, then relax down again. Keep the body steady and do not swing the dumb-bells. Use a slow and controlled motion throughout. Repeat as required.

## Bent-Over Lateral Raise

This exercise also develops the muscles around the upper body and shoulders. It is more advanced than the previous exercise. It also looks simple, yet can be quite demanding. Take care not to overload the muscles by using weights that are too heavy. Perform this exercise by starting off with holding the dumb-bells hanging in front of you, while standing bent over with knees slightly bent. Your arms should be almost straight. Lift your arms out to your sides, keeping the elbows only slightly bent throughout the motion. Do not be tempted to swing the dumb-bells, or to perform this exercise too quickly. The rest of your body should remain stationary throughout the exercise. Aim to lift the weights so that they are in line with your shoulders at the top of the motion. This exercise should be performed with the feeling that your elbows are leading the movement rather than your hands. Take care not to hold too much tension in your neck and shoulders during this exercise.

46

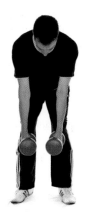

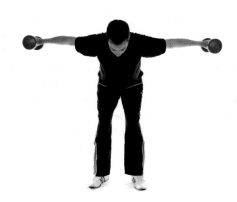

Step 1. Stand with your feet hip-width apart holding a dumb-bell in each hand. Bend the knees and look down at the ground. The dumb-bells should hang in front of you. Keep your gaze towards the ground throughout.

Step 2. Raise your arms at your sides, hold for a moment, then relax down again. Keep the body steady and do not swing the dumb-bells. Use a slow and controlled motion throughout. Repeat as required.

## Forward Lunge

This exercise targets the muscles in the legs, the quadriceps, hamstrings and the gluteals. It looks simple, yet can be quite demanding. Do not overload the muscles by using weights that are too heavy. Perform this exercise by holding the dumb-bells by your sides, with arms almost straight. They should remain stationary throughout the exercise. Take a large step forward, aiming for your front leg to be bent so that it is almost parallel to the ground. You should let your back foot come up onto the ball of the foot and also allow the back knee to bend. You will then step back and move forward with the other side.

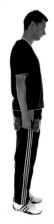

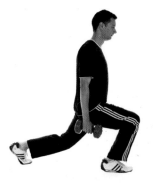

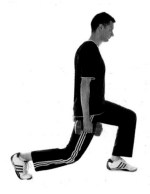

Step 1. Stand with your feet hip-width apart, holding a dumb-bell in each hand by your side.

Step 2. Take a large step forward so that your back knee bends and enables you to lower your hips. Aim for the thigh of your front leg to be parallel with the ground.

Step 3. Pull the front leg back to your starting position, then move forward using the other leg. Use a slow and controlled motion throughout. Repeat as required.

## Reverse Lunge

This exercise, like the forward lunge, targets the muscles in the legs, the quadriceps, hamstrings and the gluteals. It is an exercise that looks simple, yet can be quite demanding. Do not overload the muscles by using weights that are too heavy. Perform this exercise by starting off with holding the dumb-bells by your sides. Your arms should be almost straight and should remain stationary throughout the exercise. You will then take a large step backward. Aim for your front leg to be bent so that it is almost parallel to the ground. Let your back foot come up onto the ball of the foot and also allow the back knee to bend. Then step back up and move backward with the other side. You should aim to make as much distance going backward and you did going forward in the previous exercise.

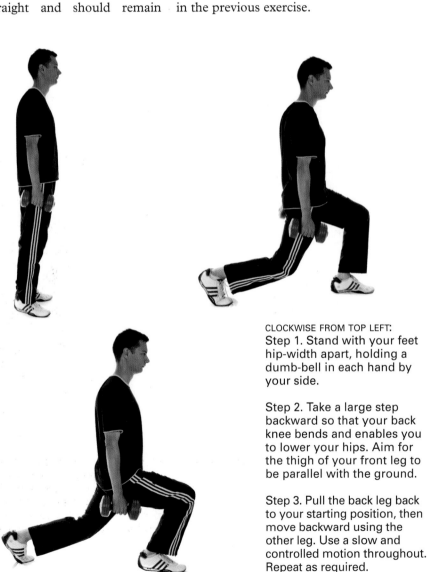

CLOCKWISE FROM TOP LEFT:
Step 1. Stand with your feet hip-width apart, holding a dumb-bell in each hand by your side.

Step 2. Take a large step backward so that your back knee bends and enables you to lower your hips. Aim for the thigh of your front leg to be parallel with the ground.

Step 3. Pull the back leg back to your starting position, then move backward using the other leg. Use a slow and controlled motion throughout. Repeat as required.

## Squat

This exercise targets the muscles in the legs and the lower back. It looks simple, yet can be quite demanding. The squat is regarded as one of the most efficient exercises for building strength in the lower body. Start by standing with the feet hip-width apart. You could hold your arms out in front of you to help keep your back as upright as possible during the exercise. You then lower the body by bending at the knees. This exercise can be made more challenging by the addition of free weights. You may feel that your ankles stop you achieving a deep squat. In this case, it will be necessary to work on developing ankle flexibility.

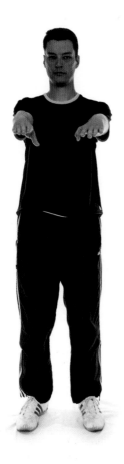

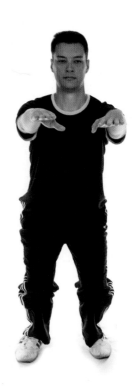

Step 1. Stand with your feet hip-width apart and your arms out in front of you.

Step 2. Bend your knees while keeping your feet flat on the ground and squat as deeply as you are comfortable with. Hold for a moment, then relax up to the starting position in Step 1. Use a slow and controlled motion throughout. Repeat as required.

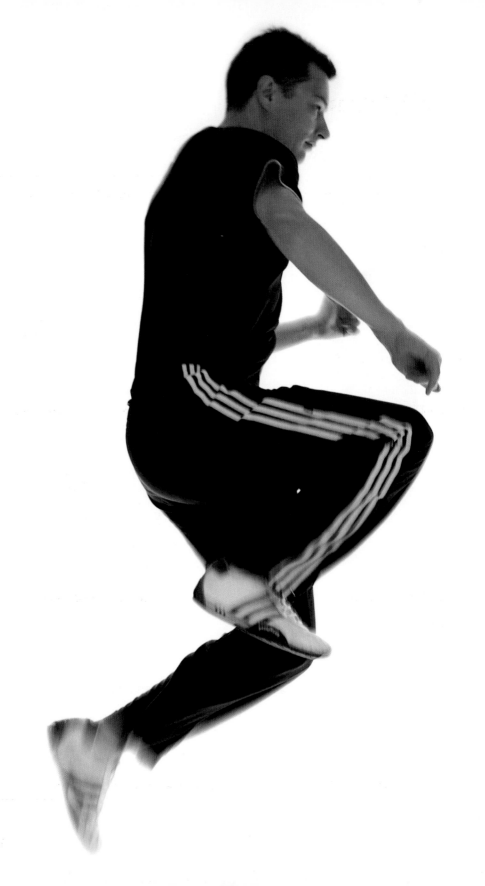

# 5    Plyometrics

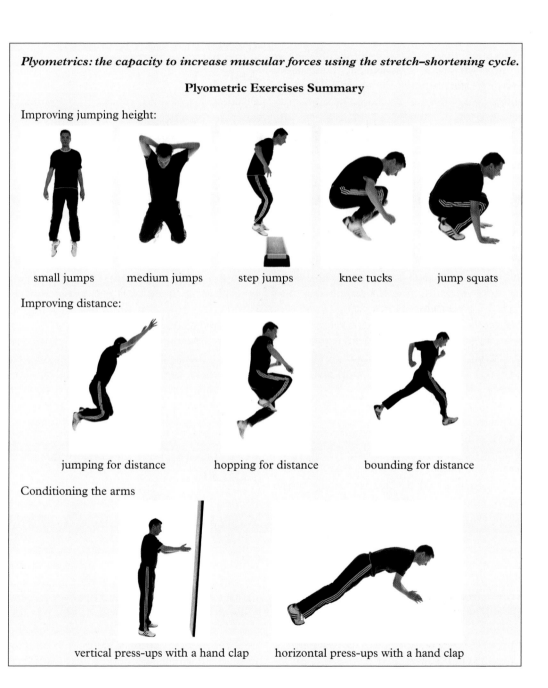

*Plyometrics: the capacity to increase muscular forces using the stretch–shortening cycle.*

**Plyometric Exercises Summary**

Improving jumping height:

small jumps          medium jumps          step jumps          knee tucks          jump squats

Improving distance:

jumping for distance          hopping for distance          bounding for distance

Conditioning the arms

vertical press-ups with a hand clap          horizontal press-ups with a hand clap

## ABOUT PLYOMETRICS

Plyometric exercises focus on increasing power. The power training in the previous chapter focused on using exercises with resistance and performing repetitions in quick succession. In plyometric training, the muscle is first stretched, then quickly contracted. Here, the time between the stretching and the shortening of the muscle should be as short as possible. This action is known as the stretch–shortening cycle. Normally, plyometric training is sport-specific, in that the exercises are designed to improve power for a movement which is typical of that particular sport. A sports coach would normally study a movement, then work on developing a drill that would help the athlete to practise correct technique and build plyometric ability. Through such training the athlete would be aiming to jump higher or further, hit harder or move faster. Improved strength may also be a by-product of such training. Examples include learning to punch with more power, or to strike a shuttlecock in badminton more effectively using forearm rotation movement.

Three common stages of a plyometric exercise can be identified:

• muscle lengthening
• short pause
• explosive muscle contraction.

Each action would be practised many times. Such repetitive training is thought to develop the muscles to work efficiently and to contract strongly and as quickly as possible within a specific movement. There are three components of plyometric movement:

• muscular power component: this is a combination of muscular strength and speed
• muscle stretch–shortening component: a muscle that is stretched before a contraction will produce a greater force through the storage of elastic energy
• neurological component: training the stretch–shortening cycle of a muscle is believed to affect its neurological response.

## BENEFITS OF TRAINING FOR PLYOMETRIC ABILITY

Plyometric training should gradually increase the efficiency of the neuromuscular connections between the brain and a trained muscle. There are other training methods that can be used to build power and strength, like those in the previous chapter. However, plyometric training is particularly useful when specific movements such as jumping and striking are involved. Much of the energy that is used in stretching the muscle is lost as heat; however, a certain amount is stored as elastic energy which can be utilized in the subsequent contraction. It is for this reason that the muscle should be contracted as quickly as possible.

Many athletes use plyometric training for activities such as long and high jumps, hurdles and throwing and hitting actions. Footballers, track and field athletes, martial artists and those involved in racket sports, for example, could benefit from such training.

## IMPROVING PLYOMETRIC ABILITY

As with any workout, you should start with a warm-up. This would typically include jogging and movement around the joints that will be involved in the plyometric exercises. A cool-down period should be included at the end of each workout. This would typically include static stretching and light movement around the joints exercised during the workout. Plyometric exercises are generally only recommended for athletes who already have a thorough grounding in resistance training. This is because plyometric exercises are considered high risk for injury and as such should only be attempted when the athlete is considered to be in good shape.

As with any exercise programme, you should start slowly and aim to build it up at a rate appropriate to your development. You should start with, say, ten repetitions, then add an extra five or ten when you are ready. The emphasis during plyometric training should be on the quality of the movement rather than the quantity. While you perform these exercises, try to be aware of where the stretch–shortening cycle occurs, how smooth your body movement is and how you are developing the effectiveness of utilizing the stretch–shortening cycle. With practice, you should be able to feel an improvement in the quality and power of the movement. Further information can be found in Chu (1998) and Radcliffe and Farentinos (1999).

## SAFETY CONSIDERATIONS

Plyometric exercises are considered to be high risk due to the nature of the movement. Such training is normally only recommended for well-conditioned athletes who have a good grounding in resistance training and even then only under supervision. For this reason, attention should be paid to the technique used and also to ensure that enough rest is built into any training programme to limit any muscular problems or injuries. For any exercises that involve impact with the ground, ensure that surfaces which provide cushioning are used, such as sprung floors in gyms and mats. You should also ensure that your trainers have a reasonable amount of cushioning built into them, so that they provide you with appropriate support. Athletes should pay particular attention to any skeletal or muscular problems that they may have and consult an appropriate medical professional before attempting such training. In any jumping exercises, care should be

taken to land in such a way that there is no undue twisting motion forced onto the joints. You should aim to land lightly on your feet, in order to minimize the impact on your body. Flexibility training is often combined with plyometric training. This can help to condition the muscles so that they are less likely to suffer from an injury.

## PLYOMETRIC EXERCISES

There are numerous sport-specific plyometric training exercises. This chapter introduces some more general developmental exercises, as a way of beginning to get a better understanding of the stretch–shortening cycle and the potential benefits of such training. This, hopefully, should make it easier to understand how such training may be applied to your specific sport. There are three types of exercises in this chapter:

• improving jumping height exercises
• improving distance exercises
• conditioning the arms exercises.

---

**Tips for the Jumping Exercises**

During the jump, aim to keep your gaze forward. You want to land firmly on both of your feet at the same time and be in a balanced position, so that you or your arms do not wobble about on landing. You can check that you land on both of your feet at the same time by listening to the sound your feet make on landing. If you hear only one sound, then you are landing with both feet at the same time. If you hear two sounds, your feet are contacting the ground at different times. This exercise is best performed in a hall or other clear area where you have enough space to perform the action. Ensure that there are no obstructions that would form a safety hazard. If you feel unbalanced, try jumping alongside a wall, so that you can quickly support yourself if need be.

---

## Small Jumps

This is the first in a series of exercises designed to work on your jump height. It is a simple exercise, suitable for starting with, and involves only a small amount of movement. With your feet hip-width apart, you perform a small jump using only your lower legs, such that you do not bend too much at the knees. Try to keep your back straight and upright throughout the movement, so that the work done during the jump mostly takes place in the feet and the calves. You should aim to increase the height of your jump as you practise. Start slowly, then when you are comfortable try to speed up as you perform the repetitions. The stretch cycle occurs while you are in the air and the explosive shortening cycle occurs while you are momentarily in contact with the ground and then pushing off for the next jump. This exercise involves impact with the ground, so ensure you are training on a suitable surface.

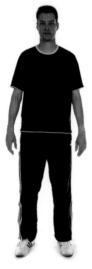

Step 1. Stand in a relaxed position with your feet hip-width apart and firmly on the ground. Keep your arms by your side.

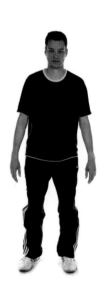

Step 2. Prepare for the jump by slightly bending your knees.

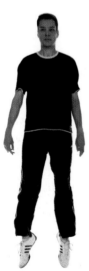

Step 3. Slowly perform a jump. Remember to land firmly on both of your feet, such that they touch the ground at the same time. Keep your back straight and upright throughout the movement. Repeat as required.

## Medium Jumps

This is the second in a series of exercises designed to work on your jump height. It is another simple exercise, but involves a larger motion than the previous exercise. With your feet hip-width apart, you perform a jump, this time bending your knees more and raising your arms above your head to help you gain height. Try to keep your back straight and upright throughout the movement so that the work done during the jump mostly takes place in the legs. You should aim to increase the height of your jump as you practice. Start slowly, then when you are comfortable try to speed up as you perform the repetitions. The stretch cycle occurs while you are in the air and the explosive shortening cycle occurs while you are momentarily in contact with the ground and then pushing off for the next jump. This exercise involves impact with the ground, so ensure that you are training on a suitable surface.

Step 1. Stand in a relaxed position with your feet hip-width apart and firmly on the ground. Keep your arms by your side.

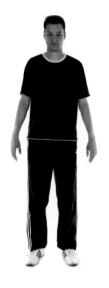

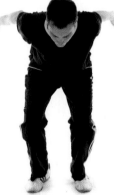

Step 2. Get your arms in a ready position to help you with the jump. Bend at the knees.

Step 3. Slowly perform a jump using your arms to help you gain height. Remember to land firmly on both of your feet, such that they touch the ground at the same time. Keep your back straight and upright throughout the movement. Repeat as required.

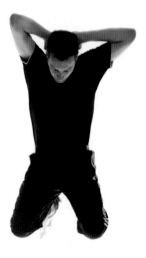

## Step Jumps

This is the third in a series of exercises designed to work on your jump height. It is a more demanding exercise than the previous two. With your feet hip-width apart, you perform a jump, but this time you will be jumping off and onto a step. You can bend your knees to help you to gain height. Try to keep your back straight and upright throughout the movement so that the work done during the jump mostly takes place in the legs and the abdomen. You should aim to increase the height of your jump as you practise. Start slowly, then when you are comfortable try speeding up as you perform the repetitions. For safety, ensure that the step is on a suitable surface and that it is stable enough to support you appropriately throughout the exercise. The stretch cycle occurs while you are in the air and the explosive shortening cycle occurs while you are momentarily in contact with the ground and then pushing off for the next jump. This exercise involves impact with the ground, so ensure that you are training on a suitable surface.

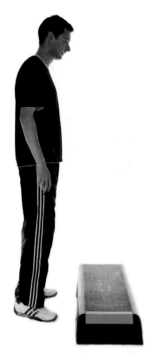 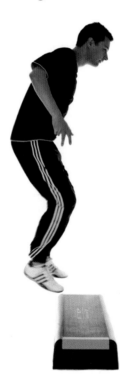 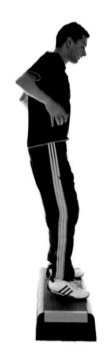

Step 1. Stand in a relaxed position with your feet hip-width apart and firmly on the ground. You should be close enough to the step to be able to comfortably and safely jump onto it. Keep your arms by your side.

Step 2. Jump up onto the step.

Step 3. Remember to land firmly on both of your feet, such that they make contact with the step at the same time. Jump down again onto the ground. Again, remember to land firmly on both of your feet, such that they make contact with the ground at the same time. Repeat as required.

## Knee Tucks

This is the fourth in a series of exercises designed to work on your jump height. It is a relatively difficult exercise compared to the previous three. With your feet hip-width apart, you perform a jump. You can bend your knees to help you to gain height. Keep your back straight and upright throughout the movement, so that the work done during the jump mostly takes place in the legs and the abdomen. This time when you jump, lift your knees as close to your chest as possible. You should aim to increase the height of your jump as you practise. Start slowly, then when you are comfortable try to speed up as you perform the repetitions. The stretch cycle occurs while you are in the air and the explosive shortening cycle occurs while you are momentarily in contact with the ground and then pushing off for the next jump. This exercise involves impact with the ground, so ensure that you are training on a suitable surface.

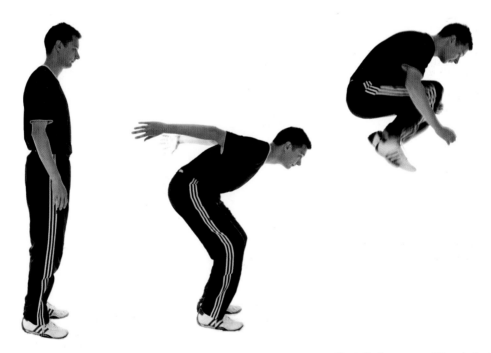

Step 1. Stand in a relaxed position with your feet hip-width apart and firmly on the ground. Keep your arms by your side.

Step 2. Prepare for the jump and the knee tuck by bending your knees and readying your arms.

Step 3. Jump up. Remember to bring your knees up high and as close to your chest as possible. Then land firmly on both of your feet, such that they touch the ground at the same time. Repeat as required.

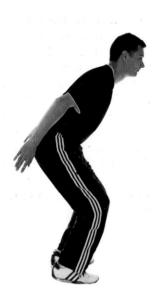

Step 1. Stand in a relaxed position with your feet hip-width apart and firmly on the ground. Prepare your arms to help you gain height.

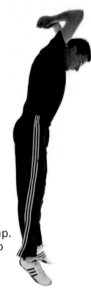

Step 2. Perform a jump. Use your arms to help you gain height.

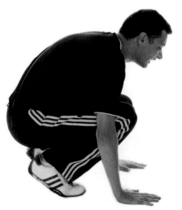

Step 3. Squat down low. Remember to land firmly on both of your feet, such that they touch the ground at the same time. Repeat as required.

## Jump Squats

This is the fifth in a series of exercises designed to work on your jump height. This is a relatively difficult exercise compared to the previous four. With your feet hip-width apart, you perform a jump. You can bend your knees to help you to gain height and you can also raise your arms above your head to help you to reach as high as possible. Keep your back straight and upright throughout the movement so that the work done during the jump mostly takes place in the legs and abdomen.

Once you land, you want to go into a quick and deep squat before jumping back up. Aim to increase the height of your jump as you practise. Start slowly, then when you are comfortable try to speed up as you perform the repetitions. The stretch cycle occurs while you are in the air and the explosive shortening cycle occurs while you are momentarily in contact with the ground and then pushing off for the next jump. This exercise involves impact with the ground, so ensure that you are training on a suitable surface.

## Jumping for Distance

This is a simple exercise, suitable for starting with if you are interested in improving your jump distance. This exercise uses a standing start and focuses on improving the jump distance rather than the jump height. With your feet hip-width apart, you perform a jump, trying to make as much horizontal distance as possible. Start off slowly so that you have time to get used to the motion involved in the exercise. Once you are comfortable with the movement, you could increase the difficulty of this exercise by increasing the distance of the jump and decreasing the time taken between jumps. You could also consider adding a short run in advance of the jump in order to improve the distance achieved during the jump. The stretch cycle occurs while you are in the air and the explosive shortening cycle occurs while you are momentarily in contact with the ground and then pushing off for the next jump. This exercise involves impact with the ground, so ensure that you are training on a suitable surface.

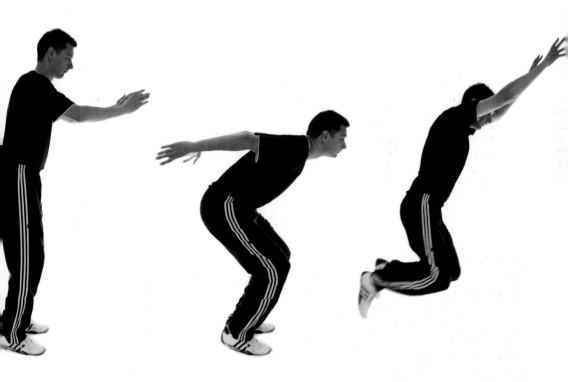

Step 1. Stand in a relaxed position with your feet hip-width apart and firmly on the ground.

Step 2. Prepare your arms ready to jump.

Step 3. Slowly perform a jump moving forward, using your arms to help you make distance.

## Hopping for Distance

This is another simple exercise to get started with if you are interested in improving your hopping distance. This exercise uses a standing start and focuses on improving the hopping distance rather than the hopping height. With one foot raised off the ground, you perform a hop, trying to make as much horizontal distance as possible. Start off slowly so that you have time to get used to the motion involved in the exercise. Once you are comfortable with the movement, you could increase the difficulty of this exercise by increasing the distance of the hop and decreasing the time between hops. The stretch cycle occurs while you are in the air and the explosive shortening cycle occurs while you are momentarily in contact with the ground and then pushing off for the next hop. This exercise involves impact with the ground, so you should ensure that you are training on a suitable surface.

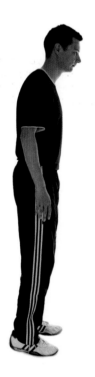 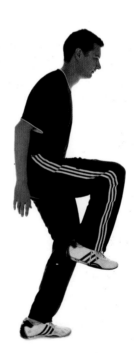 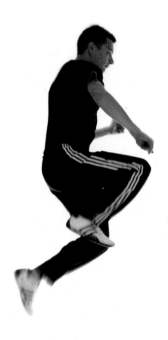

Step 1. Stand in a relaxed position with your feet hip-width apart and firmly on the ground.

Step 2. Slowly raise one leg off the floor. Do not let it touch your other leg. Adjust the height of your raised leg to suit your ability level. Once in position, focus on maintaining balance.

Step 3. Slowly perform a hop. Remember that you want to land firmly on your foot. Repeat as required.

## Bounding for Distance

This is an excellent exercise if you are interested in working on improving the distance of your movement. Bounding is basically where you perform running but with longer strides during which you try to stay in the air for as long as possible. The stretch cycle occurs while you are in the air and the explosive shortening cycle occurs as you contact and then push off the ground into the next bound. This exercise is best performed in a clear area. You could make this exercise easy to start off with by trying it out slowly. Once you are comfortable with the movement, you could work on building up the speed. You could consider modifying this exercise as you develop by increasing the vertical component of your movement as well as the horizontal component. This exercise involves impact with the ground and, so you ensure that you are training on a suitable surface.

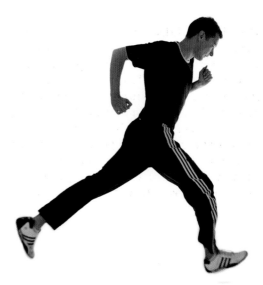

Stand in a relaxed position with your feet hip-width apart and firmly on the ground. Start to run forward and steadily build up your stride length and the time spent in the air. Repeat as required.

## Vertical Press-Ups with a Hand Clap

This exercise is a good starter for conditioning your arms for plyometric exercise. It starts in the press-up position, but standing up rather than being on the ground. Start by positioning yourself a couple of feet away from a wall, then placing your hands on the wall in front so that you are leaning forward. You then perform a press-up and when you are almost standing straight in the movement, clap your hands. Continue on into the next press up. You can build on this exercise by increasing the speed at which you do it. If you find this exercise too easy, try the next one, which is the same exercise but starts in the normal, horizontal press-up position. The stretch cycle occurs during the movement where your hands are off the wall. The explosive shortening action occurs during the contact with the wall and backward motion when you push off the wall to enable you to clap. Aim keep your contact time with the wall and the time between press-ups as short as possible.

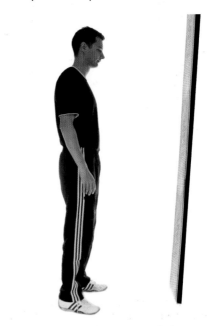

Step 1. Stand in a relaxed position with your feet hip-width apart and firmly on the ground. You should be about 2ft (60cm) away from the wall.

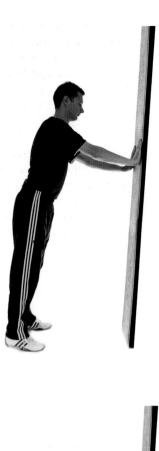

LEFT: Step 2. Place your palms on the wall directly in front of you. Ensure that your body remains straight, such that you are not bending at the waist to reach the wall.

BELOW: Step 3. Perform a press-up off the wall.

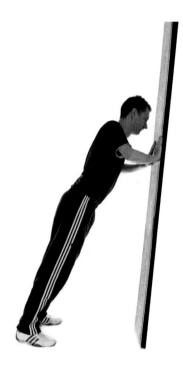

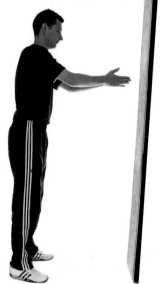

Step 4. Then clap your hands as you move away from the wall. Move into the position in Step 2 again so that you are ready for the next press-up. Repeat as required.

## Horizontal Press-Ups with a Hand Clap

This exercise is a more advanced version of the previous one. It combines a proper press-up with a hand clap, so it is quite demanding in terms of upper body strength. Do not attempt this exercise if you are not able to perform press-ups easily. This exercise starts in the standard press-up position on the ground. Ensure that your palms are firmly on the ground and directly under your shoulders. Also, ensure that your body remains straight during the press-up, for example do not bend at the waist or in your back. You then perform a press-up and when you are moving upwards, you clap your hands. Then you continue on into the next press-up. You can build on this exercise by increasing the speed at which you do it. The stretch cycle occurs during the movement where your hands are off the ground. The explosive shortening action occurs during the contact with the ground and the backward motion when you push off the ground to enable you to clap. Aim to keep your contact time with the ground and the time between press-ups as short as possible.

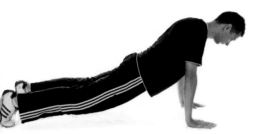

Step 1. Start in the standard press-up position, with your body straight. Your palms should be firmly on the ground and directly beneath your shoulders.

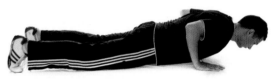

Step 2. Perform a press-up.

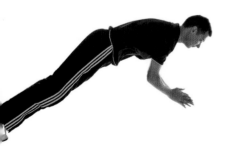

Step 3. Clap your hands as you move away from the ground.

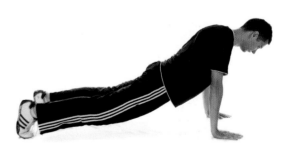

Step 4. Move into the position in Step 1 again so that you are ready for the next press-up. Repeat as required.

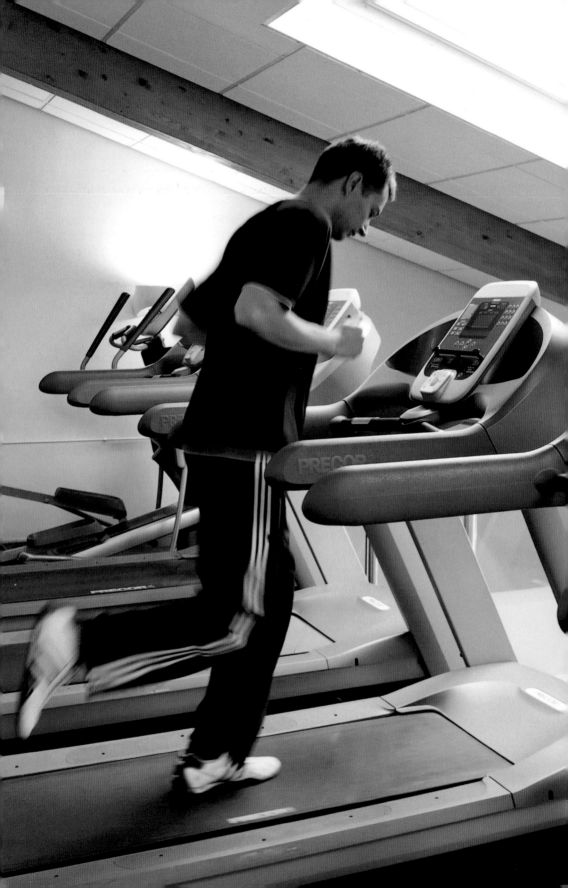

# 6    Stamina

*Stamina: the capacity to sustain low-level aerobic work for a long period of time.*

**Stamina Exercises Summary**

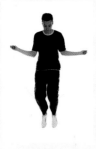 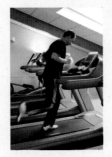 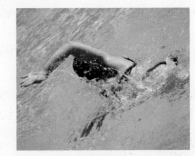

skipping            jogging            swimming

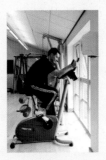 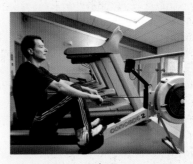

cycling            rowing

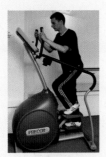 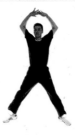

stair climbing       star jump and press-up combination

# ABOUT STAMINA

Stamina is the ability to sustain prolonged activity. This is often also called endurance. The definition of what is prolonged activity is dependent on the type of exercise that is under consideration, so it can mean minutes, hours or even days. Endurance training normally consists of a sustained activity such as jogging, swimming, cycling or skipping for extended amounts of time. The focus is on building up the length of time that the activity can be sustained through repeated training sessions.

# BENEFITS OF TRAINING FOR STAMINA

Stamina training can improve the effectiveness of the lungs and heart and improve the health of the blood vessels. This in turn can lead to a decreased risk of heart attacks, strokes and other diseases that are caused by a weak heart.

Stamina training will help you to carry out everyday tasks that require endurance more effectively, such as running to catch a train, climbing up stairs and hill walking. Overall, it should make it easier to maintain a more active lifestyle. If you are involved in sports, then endurance training will help you to keep going for longer. This is of vital importance in sports such as football, rugby, tennis, long-distance running and long-distance swimming. Some form of endurance training is normally recommended as part of a healthy lifestyle and as an accompaniment for many sports. However, stamina training alone will not help to combat muscle loss due to aging. Stamina training is not a substitute for strength training.

# IMPROVING STAMINA

Stamina is built up gradually by taking the body through repeated training with suffi-

cient rest periods between training. You could start by attempting five minutes of an exercise, then once you can comfortably achieve that you could try adding another five minutes of training. Your aim is to, over time, build up your stamina and therefore the amount of time that you can keep going. Such training will inevitably result in an increased heart and breathing rate. Once you have settled into such training, it is better to attempt each exercise for a minimum of twenty minutes, so that your body has time to start getting into aerobic activity. Ideally, stamina training should be incorporated into your routine as often as possible. A good target would be to try some every other day. Remember that it does not have to be the same exercise each time. Variety could be added to your training programme by doing a different activity in each session, so that you rotate through the activity types. Jogging, cycling, skipping, swimming, walking briskly and hill walking are all ways in which you can build up your endurance. If, however, you find that you prefer one form of endurance training, then it is better to stick to that than to not do any training at all. These exercises can also be used in the form of a light warm-up activity as a prelude to other training. Further information can be found in Ackland (2007), Radcliffe and Farentinos (1999) and Kahn and Biscontini (2006).

# SAFETY CONSIDERATIONS

Since endurance training can be hard work for your heart, you should be particularly aware of stopping exercise if you experience any of the following:

• breathing difficulties
• dizziness
• chest pain.

Where safety equipment is available, for example cycle helmets and glow-in-the-dark strips, ensure that you use them. If you decide to jog or run, suitable footwear is vital. Stretching after a workout will help to reduce post-training muscle soreness. Also, ensure that you warm up and cool down as part of your stamina workout.

## STAMINA EXERCISES

### Skipping
This is an exercise that requires little space when compared to the other exercises in this chapter. You will need a skipping rope for this activity. You could start off by trying to skip for a couple of minutes without taking any breaks. Once you are able to complete that, you could build up to a complete five minutes of skipping. Once five minutes gets too easy, steadily build up to twenty to thirty minutes of skipping. You could start by skipping with your feet together using a jumping action. Once you are comfortable with this, try different footwork combinations as a way of keeping you interested and challenged.

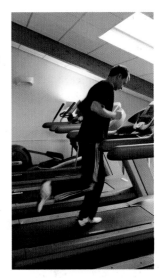

Jogging is a stamina exercise that can be done outdoors or even within in a gym on a running machine.

### Jogging
Suitable footwear is vital, particularly if you will be jogging on surfaces that are hard, like pavements or floors that are not sprung. If you are not used to jogging, you are likely to find it particularly difficult. You may want to start off with a simpler version of jogging, in which you jog on the spot and slowly try to build up the time that you are able to continue the activity. Once you feel that jogging on the spot is easy, try jogging in the park, in a hall or on a track. Remember to give yourself time to build up the activity. If you have not been jogging properly for a long time, then even a few minutes might be more than you can manage. You will need to give your body time to develop to be able to cope with greater exertion. You could carry out this type of exercise in a gym on a running machine.

### Swimming
Swimming is an excellent low-impact way of training for endurance. However, it is also likely to be an expensive way to train. Swimming is normally ideal if you are worried about any muscular or skeletal problems. There are a number of different

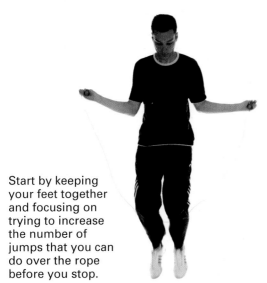

Start by keeping your feet together and focusing on trying to increase the number of jumps that you can do over the rope before you stop.

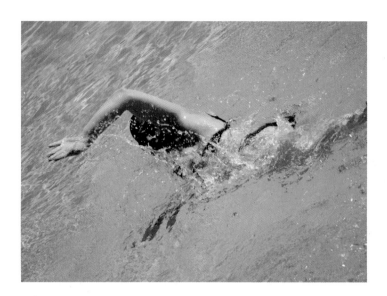

Swimming can be an excellent low-impact form of stamina training.

swimming strokes that you could try, for example front crawl or breast stroke. With swimming, like all stamina-building activities, you will need to be patient with your development. If you are not used to swimming, you are likely to find it difficult to swim many laps without stopping, However, if you continue to practise, you should start to find it easier to do the laps faster and to do more of them over time without needing a break. Swimming does not need to be done for hours on end. It is better to start with five minutes of a good workout, then try to build that up to fifteen or twenty minutes. Certainly, if you manage to swim non-stop for thirty minutes at a reasonable pace, you are doing quite well and should focus on improving your swimming speed so that you complete more laps in less time.

## Cycling

Cycling is another type of exercise that you could use to build your stamina. You will need either a bicycle or a cycling machine like the ones available in gyms. A good way of continuing cycling training is to make it part of your everyday routine. For example,

if you work close enough to home, you could consider cycling to work, or you could perhaps make cycling part of the way that you take trips at the weekend. If you will be cycling outdoors, ensure that you use all the appropriate safety equipment.

## Rowing

Rowing is another form of stamina training. It works all of the major muscles in the body and so makes it an excellent form of exercise. Many gyms have rowing machines, which can make it an accessible form of exercise. If you plan to row, either outdoors or in a gym, ensure that you train under supervision as poor technique can lead to injuries, including back pain.

## Stair Climbing

Going up the stairs can be a very good form of stamina training. You could make a conscious effort to take the stairs instead of using lifts and escalators. Steps are also used in step aerobics and gyms often have step machines that can be fairly easily accessed for training. You should wear suitable footwear to minimize the impact on your joints.

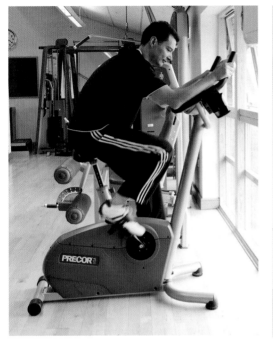

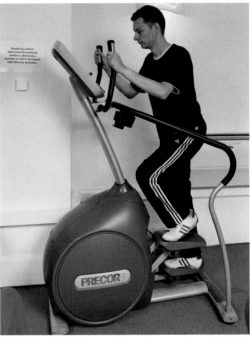

Cycling is a stamina exercise that can be done outdoors or within in a gym on a cycling machine.

Step machines can be used for developing stamina.

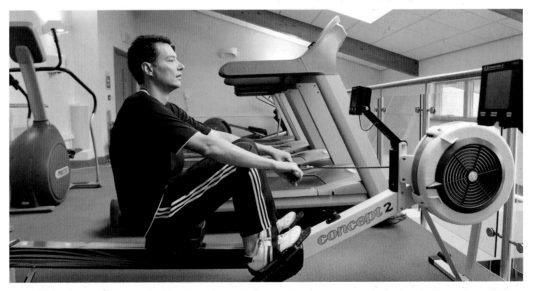

Rowing is a stamina exercise that can be done outdoors or even within in a gym on a rowing machine.

STRATHFIELD MUNICIPAL LIBRARY

## Star Jump and Press-Up Combination

If you lack space but still wish to train indoors, this exercise is appropriate for you. It requires no equipment and little space.

This exercise may sound easy, but it is in fact demanding and very tiring. Start off with sets of five and build it up slowly over time. Ensure that you wear suitable footwear to reduce any impact on your joints.

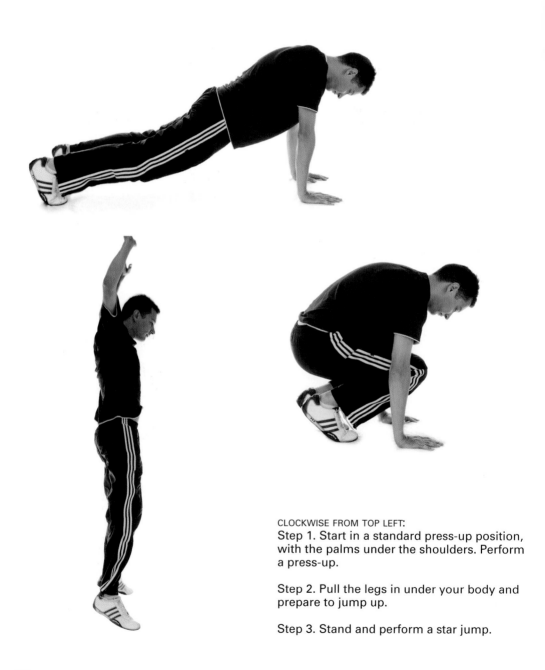

CLOCKWISE FROM TOP LEFT:
Step 1. Start in a standard press-up position, with the palms under the shoulders. Perform a press-up.

Step 2. Pull the legs in under your body and prepare to jump up.

Step 3. Stand and perform a star jump.

Step 4. Come back down into the position in Step 2.

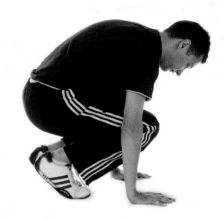

Step 5. Push the legs back out into the press-up position and complete a press-up. Repeat as required.

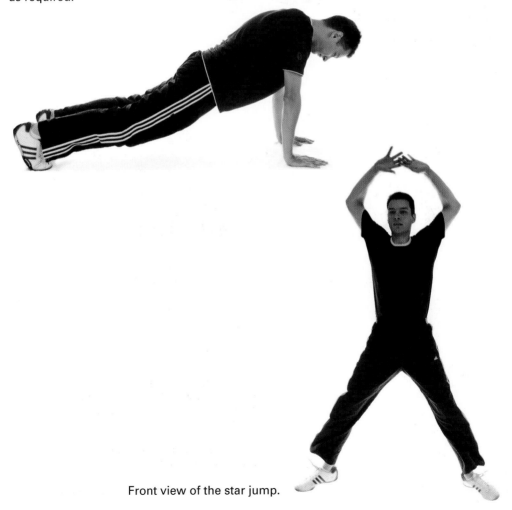

Front view of the star jump.

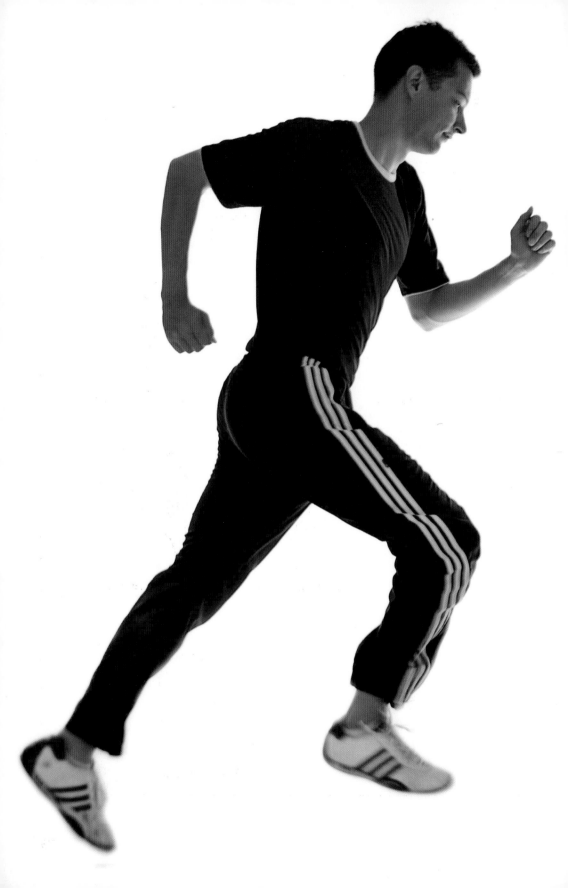

# 7    Speed

*Speed: the capacity to move the whole body or limbs quickly.*

## Speed Exercises Summary

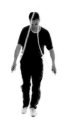

skipping with alternating feet

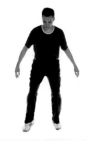

jumping in and out

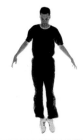

jumping side to side

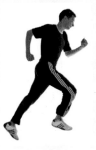

running

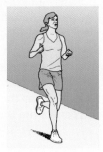

running downhill

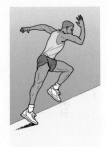

running uphill

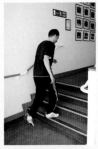

running up steps

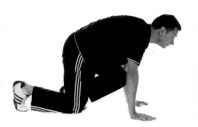

acceleration exercises

# ABOUT SPEED

Speed training is about increasing the speed at which you can move or perform a particular action. Speed is often an important part of any sport. An athlete's speed is influenced by their ability to move, as well as their strength and technique. Speed training often involves the initial training of the body with good technique in slow motion. Then the body needs to practise performing good technique at faster and faster speeds. This is in order to get the body trained into moving correctly and efficiently at high speeds. Any inefficiencies in the movement can lead to decreased speed.

Speed training should normally be done when the muscles are not in a condition of fatigue. A good warm-up and appropriate flexibility training should help to improve performance. The development of muscular strength should also help to improve speed performance. Normally, speed training exercises will involve slow-motion technique training accompanied by much faster and shorter interval high-speed actions. This form of training is believed to improve the firing of the correct muscular response.

# BENEFITS OF TRAINING FOR SPEED

There are a number of things that a speed training programme looks to achieve:

• improving acceleration
• improving maximum velocity
• increasing the time before fatigue sets in.

The last point, improving the time before muscle fatigue sets in, can be improved through strength endurance training. The explosive nature of plyometric training can also help to develop maximum velocity and acceleration. When speed training also involves a change in direction, this is normally termed agility training. This is covered separately in the next chapter.

# IMPROVING SPEED

Speed training requires the brain and nervous system to work more effectively at getting the muscles to contract quicker for the completion of the movement. To be most effective, speed training should be carried out throughout the year, so that the brain does not have to relearn the control over the muscles when speed is required. It is all to do with the brain learning effective muscle control patterns and being able to utilize them at the right time. Appropriate rest and recovery periods need to be incorporated into any speed training programme. With running speed, you would be looking to improve the stride length and stride frequency. Any other training that is performed during a speed training programme should be of low intensity so that the body is not too fatigued to benefit from the speed activities.

If you are preparing for an event, you want to aim to do shorter runs at a speed faster than the average speed you are aiming for in the event. This should help to develop stamina at your desired speed. Initially, you should allow long recovery periods, then as your training progresses it should be possible to reduce your recovery periods. It is useful to have a stopwatch for use in speed training, as this will enable you to track any improvements in your run times. If you keep a record of your achievements over time, you should be able to get a sense of how you are developing. Further information can be found in Ward and Dintiman (2003) and Smith (2005).

# SAFETY CONSIDERATIONS

Since speed training involves fast movements and footwork, it is advisable to wear appropriate footwear and also to train on a suitable surface. Speed training is best carried out when the body is not fatigued. During speed training it can be easy to forget that good technique should be used with each movement. If you find that you start to use bad technique, slow down to introduce back in the good technique before speeding up again. This should help to reduce the risk of injury.

# SPEED EXERCISES

### Skipping with Alternating Feet
Skipping is a good way of developing fast and coordinated footwork. Performing skipping exercises fast and for increasing lengths of time will encourage you to develop your technique and minimize any unwanted movements that slow you down. For example, if you are looking to jump over the rope faster and faster, you will need to decrease how high you jump over the rope so that you can make contact with the ground faster before the rope comes around again. You should begin to find that your feet barely come off the ground the faster that you attempt this exercise. Also, ensuring that your feet work together, in that they impact the ground at the same time, will enable you to keep going for longer, without tripping up the rope and having to stop. The beneficial thing about skipping is that, unlike running, it does not require much space and certainly does not cost much money. In addition, as well as developing fast footwork, you will be able to use this form of exercise for stamina training as well improving your coordination.

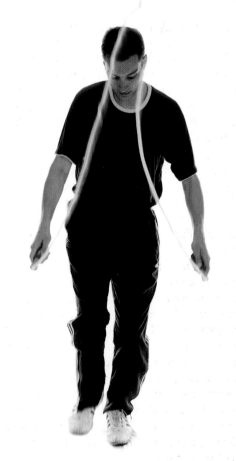

Skipping while jumping over the rope using alternating feet is a good way to develop speed and fast footwork. In addition, it will improve you coordination and your technique.

Once you are able to jump quickly while using both feet together, you could then try jumping over the rope using alternating feet. This will feel much more like a running motion, but will require even greater coordination and technique in order to build up the speed and reduce the number of times that you trip up on the rope. This exercise can be quite high impact, so you should wear suitable footwear and train on a suitable surface.

## Jumping In and Out

This is another exercise that is often used to develop fast feet. Here you start in a position with your feet together. You then jump forward, but land with your feet hip-width apart. From here, jump forward again and land with your feet together. You can use this sequence to jump along a line in a hall and work on building up your speed as you go. The focus in this exercise on how quickly you can land and then spring back into the next jump. Also, in order to improve speed you will need to focus on decreasing any unwanted motion. For example, you could aim to reduce the vertical component of your jump as much as possible each time and focus on improving the horizontal distance. In this way, a combination of jump speed and jump length is employed to improve the time in which you can complete a certain distance. This exercise can be quite high impact, so you should wear suitable footwear and train on an appropriate surface.

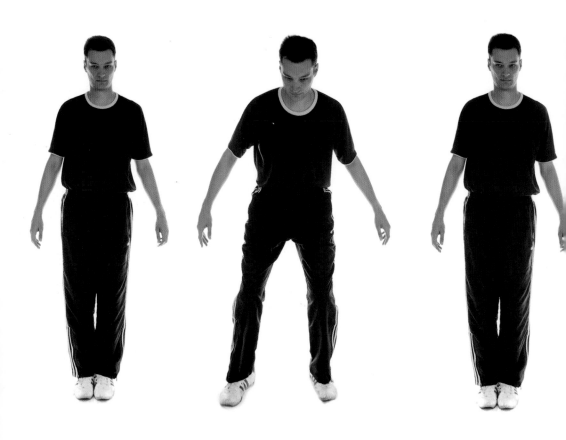

Step 1. Stand to one side with both of your feet together.

Step 2. Jump forward and land with your feet hip-width apart.

Step 3. Jump forward and land with your feet together. Repeat this sequence as required.

**Jumping Side to Side**

This is another exercise that is often used to develop fast feet. Here you start in a position with your feet together, then jump to the side and slightly forward, landing with your feet together. From here, you jump to the other side and slightly forward again, landing with your feet together. You can use this sequence to jump along a line in a hall and work on building up your speed as you go. The focus in this exercise on how quickly you can land and then spring back into the next jump. Also, in order to improve speed you will need to focus on decreasing any unwanted motion. For example, you could aim to reduce the vertical component of your jump as much as possible each time and focus on improving the horizontal distance. In this way, you use a combination of jump speed and jump length to improve the time in which you can complete a certain distance. This exercise can be quite high impact, so you should wear suitable footwear and train on an appropriate surface.

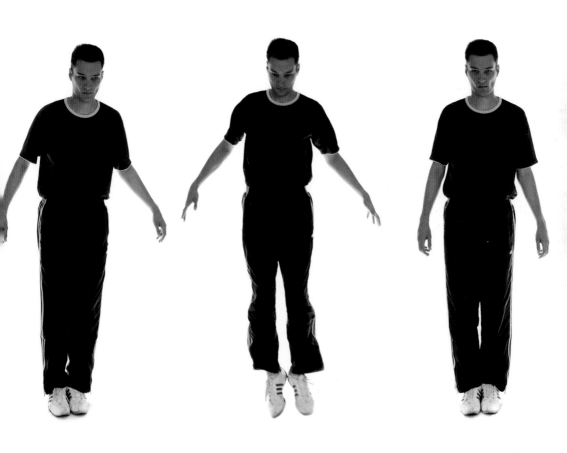

Step 1. Stand to one side with both feet together.

Step 2. Jump across to the other side and slightly forward.

Step 3. Land with your feet together. Repeat this sequence as required.

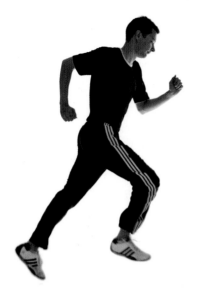

Running is a good exercise for developing speed. In addition, it will improve cardiovascular health and muscle endurance if you run for long distances.

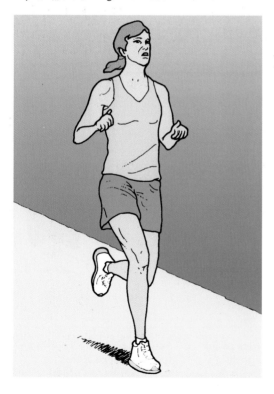

## Running

Running exercises are the most obvious ways in which to improve speed. There are a number of factors that can affect running speed including:

• stride length
• stride frequency
• acceleration
• running technique
• endurance
• distance to cover.

These are all factors on which you could focus your running in turn as you look to develop your speed and technique. In addition to developing speed, running is also a stamina exercise and will be beneficial for cardiovascular health, especially if you run for long distances. It is for this reason that running is often combined with a strength training programme as part of a healthy lifestyle. The strength training part will work towards maintaining and improving muscle strength and mass. If you are planning to run competitively, you will need to develop your running technique in order to achieve better run times. This exercise can be quite high impact, you should wear suitable footwear and train on an appropriate surface.

## Downhill Running

This is a method that can be used for developing sprinting speed. It helps to develop stride frequency, technique, acceleration and stride length. Downhill running also encourages rapid arm action. You will need to ensure that you can find a suitably safe location for carrying out such an exercise. In addition, you should ensure that the slope of the hill is not too great, as downhill running is more dangerous and carries a higher risk of injury than regular running. This exercise can be quite high impact, so you should wear suitable footwear and train on an appropriate surface.

Downhill running can be a good way to develop sprinting speed, rapid arm action, technique and acceleration.

## Uphill Running

Uphill running can also be a useful form of training and is particularly beneficial for developing running technique. This is because any side to side motion that you have will reduce your forward motion and uphill running can highlight that negative motion. Uphill running will help you to focus on your forward motion and reduce any unwanted movements that your technique may have picked up. Ensure that you find a suitably safe location for carrying out such an exercise. In addition, ensure that the slope of the hill is not too great, as uphill running can be more dangerous and carry a higher risk of injury than regular running. This exercise can be quite high impact, so you should wear suitable footwear and train on an appropriate surface.

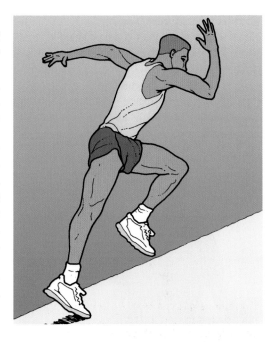

Uphill running can be used to combat any side to side action that becomes a part of your running technique. This kind of training will help to improve your forward motion and hence your overall forward speed.

## Running Up Steps

Running up the stairs is another form of speed training that is often used. Again, it is particularly beneficial for developing running technique. This is because any side to side motion that you have will reduce your forward motion and running up the stairs can highlight that negative motion. This activity will help you to focus on your forward motion and reduce any unwanted movements that your technique may have picked up. You will need to ensure that you can find a suitably safe location for carrying out such an exercise. Running up stairs can be more dangerous and carry a higher risk of injury than regular running. This exercise can be quite high impact, so you should wear suitable footwear and train on a suitable surface.

Running up steps can also be used to combat any side to side action that becomes a part of your running technique. This kind of training will help to improve your forward motion and hence your overall forward speed.

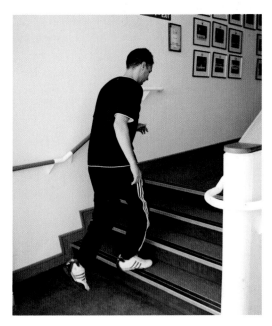

## Acceleration Exercises

These exercises focus on developing acceleration. This is done through the use of various starting positions. You can practise starting your sprints or your runs with a variety of starting positions. Once you feel that you have gained as much as you can from a particular starting position, try another one. Each different starting position will have different challenges in terms of trying to reduce the amount of movement and time required in order to get into the run. Some examples of starting positions that can be used to develop acceleration are shown here.

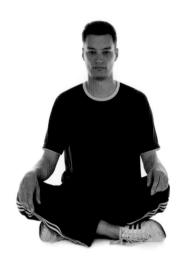

A starting position for training for acceleration: sitting cross-legged.

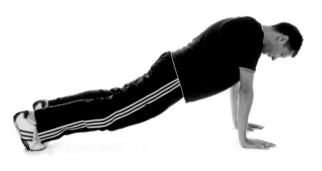

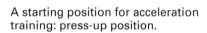

A starting position for acceleration training: press-up position.

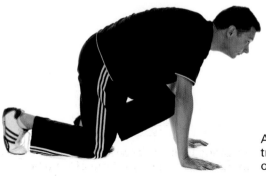

A starting position for acceleration training: on one knee with hands on the ground.

A starting position for acceleration training: on all fours.

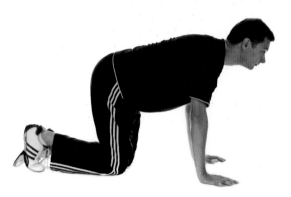

A starting position for acceleration training: sitting with both legs out in front.

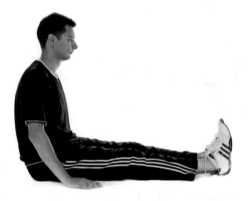

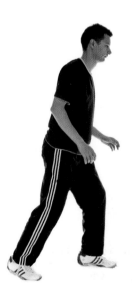

A starting position for acceleration training: standing with one leg in front of the other.

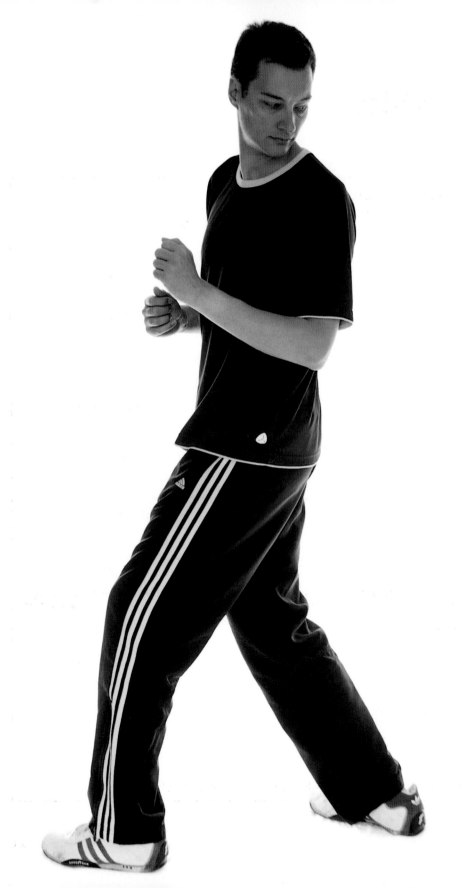

# 8    Agility

*Agility: the capacity to change direction rapidly.*

**Agility Exercises Summary**

On the spot:

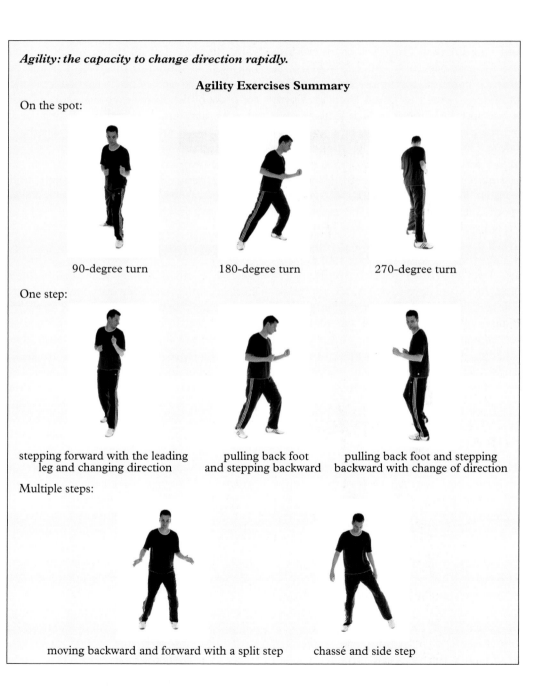

90-degree turn       180-degree turn       270-degree turn

One step:

stepping forward with the leading     pulling back foot     pulling back foot and stepping
leg and changing direction     and stepping backward     backward with change of direction

Multiple steps:

moving backward and forward with a split step       chassé and side step

# ABOUT AGILITY

Agility is the ability to change direction rapidly. This ability can be developed through improving a number of other fitness components such as strength, speed and coordination. However, there are also specific exercises that you can practise in order to improve your agility. A lot of agility training is related to speed training. There is one addition though, which is being able to change direction quickly, efficiently and safely. There are many sports that require high levels of agility, for example badminton and squash. Much agility training is normally sport- or activity-specific. However, there is no reason that these exercises cannot be used in order to develop general agility. During training, it is important to train in a safe manner and at a level that is appropriate. Agility exercises focus on developing quick footwork. There are many children's games that require agility – for example, when children are moving around a hall and are then asked to change direction when the teacher claps – and these can also be an excellent way of developing your agility.

## BENEFITS OF TRAINING FOR AGILITY

There are many sports that you can potentially take part in where a high level of agility will enhance your ability to participate at a higher standard. Good agility will also help you in everyday life to:

• avoid dangerous objects on the ground
• manoeuvre around moving objects
• complete complicated changes of direction.

Speed and good footwork together will help you to improve your agility. The exercises in this chapter will take you through types of movement and footwork that you may not be accustomed to. It should show you that there are many different ways in which you can move to achieve changes in direction. Some of these unusual footwork combinations are really useful in helping to keep your centre of gravity low and both of your feet in contact with the ground at all times, which in turn will help to minimize the risk of falling or being pushed over. This is particularly true for some of the exercises that are taken from martial arts training, where falling over would be a real disadvantage. Football, dance and racket sports are examples where good footwork is essential. Being able to move around efficiently and safely will greatly enhance your performance, whilst minimizing any risk of injury.

## IMPROVING AGILITY

There are many sports that require high levels of agility and they each have exercises appropriate for agility training. Normally, when people are training for a particular sport they will practise movements that match the types of movement they are likely to encounter in the sport. For example, in martial arts students would practise changing direction in order to be able to face opponents coming from different directions. In football, dribbling the ball requires quick changes in direction. Sports like badminton, tennis and squash require high levels of direction changing at speed in order to return the shuttlecock or the ball.

It is useful to have a stopwatch for use in agility training, as you are trying to develop the speed with which you can change direction. There are two main ways in which you could measure your agility development:

• For each exercise, keep a note of how long it takes to do a fixed number of sets. For example, how long does it take to do ten sets of a particular exercise? Then, while you continue to train, time yourself and see whether you are getting faster at being able to complete the exercise competently and safely.

- For each exercise, keep a note of how many sets you can do within a certain time. For example, how many sets of a particular exercise can you do in one minute? Then, while you continue to train, monitor your progress through the improvement in the number of sets you can achieve within a fixed amount of time.

If you keep a record of your achievements over time, then you should be able to get a sense of how you are developing. If you are planning to use these exercises for doing repetitions, you may find it useful to have some music playing in the background to help you to keep going.

You can build up your agility training by practising the exercise slowly at first and allowing your body to get used to the movement. This should help to reduce the risk of injury, while also making you aware of how your body is coping with the changes of direction. You should be particularly mindful of how your joints are coping with the movement and whether it is safe to continue. Once your body gets accustomed to the movement, you could think about starting to increase the pace at which you carry out the exercise. Another way to make the exercise a little more difficult is to try increasing the scale of the movement, for example by using bigger steps or by making the change in direction more pronounced. Further information can be found in Kielbaso (2005) and Brown and Ferrigno (2005).

## SAFETY CONSIDERATIONS

Since you will be planning to speed up your movement and the rate at which you change direction, you should ensure that the space you will be training in is free of any hazardous objects and that the floor is not slippery or unsafe in any way. Also ensure that you have protected your feet sufficiently by wearing suitable footwear. Since agility training requires working at speed and changing direction, it may put a strain on your joints, so you should ensure that you train safely and stop if you feel any discomfort. Before performing the exercises at speed, try them out slowly first. This will give you a good idea of how much space you need in which to perform them safely. Then, when you are ready, slowly build up the speed at which you attempt the exercises. Do not attempt agility exercises without medical advice, particularly if you have any muscular-skeletal problems.

## AGILITY EXERCISES

### 90-Degree Turn

This is the first of three exercises that look at making a turn using only a small amount of ground coverage. They focus on the turn rather than making any kind of distance within the movement. These exercises are based on footwork taken from karate training. In this exercise, you are trying to make a turn of 90 degrees. You will start with your left leg forward and with your arms in a fighting position. You then turn your head to look 90 degrees to your left and pull your front leg in to the centre of your body, before pushing out again in line with your gaze. You should end up in the same body position as you started in, but having turned through 90 degrees to your left. When you move your feet across the ground, focus on sliding your foot lightly along the ground rather than lifting and stepping, so as to keep both of your feet in contact with the ground throughout the movement.

Start by trying this exercise slowly, building up speed as you become more comfortable with the movement. If you can remain on the balls of your feet throughout the exercise and keep light-footed, you should find that you can complete the movement more smoothly.

You only have to lift your heel off the ground a tiny amount to be able to benefit from it. Practise this movement with either leg in the forward position.

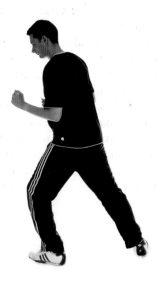

Step 1. Step forward with your left leg and stand in a relaxed fighting position. Keep up on the balls of your feet if possible.

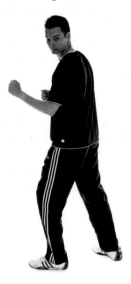

Step 2. Turn your head 90 degrees to look in the direction in which you wish to move next.

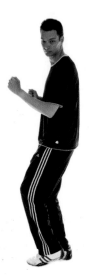

Step 3. Pull the front foot to your centre and then push it out again at 90 degrees in line with your gaze.

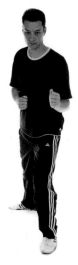

Step 4. You should be standing in the same body position as in Step 1, but now facing in a different direction. Repeat as required.

## 180-Degree Turn

This is the second of three exercises that look at making a turn using only a small amount of ground coverage. In this exercise, you are trying to make a slightly more advanced turn of 180 degrees from your starting position, so that you are then facing in the opposite direction from which you started. You start with your left leg forward and your arms in a fighting position, as in the previous exercise. You then turn your head round to your left to look behind you and pull your front leg in to the centre of your body, before pushing out again in line with your gaze. You should end up in the same body position as you started in, but having turned through 180 degrees to

your left. When you move your feet across the ground, focus on sliding your foot lightly along the ground rather than lifting and stepping, so as to keep both of your feet in contact with the ground throughout the movement.

Start by trying this exercise slowly, gradually building up speed as you become more comfortable with the movement. If you can remain on the balls of your feet throughout the exercise and keep light-footed, you should find that you can complete the movement more smoothly. You only have to lift your heel off the ground a tiny amount to be able to benefit from it. Practise this movement with either leg in the forward position.

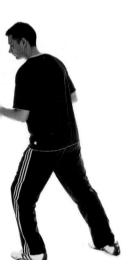
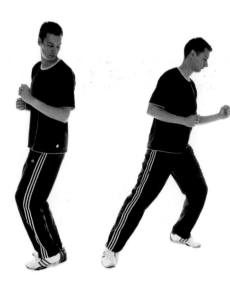

Step 1. Step forward with your left leg and stand in a relaxed fighting position.

Step 2. Turn your head round to your left to look behind you.

Step 3. Pull the front foot to your centre and then push it out again at 180 degrees.

Step 4. Turn on both feet so that you are standing in the same body position as in Step 1, but are now facing in the opposite direction. Repeat as required.

## 270-Degree Turn

This is the third of three exercises that look at making a turn using only a small amount of ground coverage. In this exercise, you are trying to make an advanced turn of 270 degrees from your starting position when moving along the outside of the leading leg. Start with your left leg forward and your arms in a fighting position, as in the previous exercise. Then turn your head round 90 degrees to your right (for a movement 270 degrees round from your left) and pull your front leg in to the centre of your body before pushing out again in line with your gaze. Your front foot will pass behind your rear foot in this motion. You should end up in the same body position as you started in, but having turned through 270 degrees to your left. When you move your feet across the ground, focus on sliding your foot lightly along the ground rather than lifting and stepping, so as to keep both of your feet in contact with the ground throughout the movement.

Start slowly, building up speed as you become more comfortable with the movement. If you can remain on the balls of your feet throughout the exercise and keep light-footed, you should find that you can complete the movement more smoothly. You only have to lift your heel off the ground a tiny amount to be able to benefit from it. Practise this movement with either leg in the forward position.

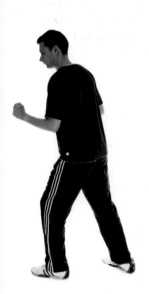 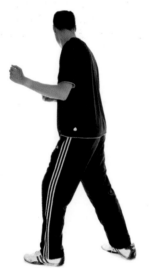 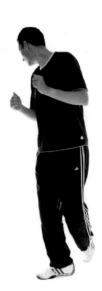 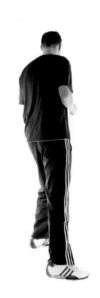

Step 1. Step forward with your left leg and stand in a relaxed fighting position.

Step 2. Turn your head to look in the direction in which you wish to move next.

Step 3. Pull the front foot to your centre, cross your back foot and then push it out again at 270 degrees.

Step 4. Then turn on both feet so that you are standing in the same body position as in Step 1 but are now facing in a different direction. Repeat as required.

## Step Forward with the Leading Leg and Change Direction

This is the first of three exercises that focuses on movement which includes a single step. Martial arts, particularly, karate and kung fu, include training in methods of moving around in order to face an opponent who is also moving freely. This leads to quite detailed training in different types of footwork. Stepping forward, then dragging the back foot in is a common method in which to make distance and also to change direction.

In this exercise, the front foot is used to lunge forward and the back foot is then lightly pulled in behind so that you are in a stable position. When you move your feet across the ground, focus on sliding your foot lightly along the ground rather than lifting and stepping, so that both feet are in contact with the ground throughout the movement. Start slowly, building up speed as you become more comfortable with the move-

ment. If you can remain on the balls of your feet throughout the exercise and keep light-footed, you should find that you can complete the movement more smoothly. You only have to lift your heel off the ground a tiny amount to be able to benefit from it. Practise this movement with either leg in the forward position.

You should practise the footwork first (Steps 1 to 4) without adding the change of direction. When you are comfortable with this footwork, continue through to Step 7, where the change of direction is added. Here you turn your head to look in the direction that you wish to move and then take your step forward in that direction. This can be a useful way in which to change direction in less than a 90-degree turn. Once you are looking to achieve bigger turns or changes in direction you would need to use the more elaborate footwork that was presented in the exercises earlier in this chapter.

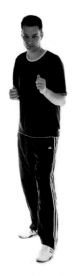 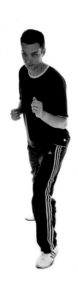 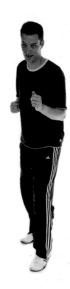

Step 1. Step forward with your left leg and stand in a relaxed fighting position.

Step 2. Take a large step forward with your left leg.

Step 3. Lightly pull the back foot in so that you are standing in the same body position as in Step 1.

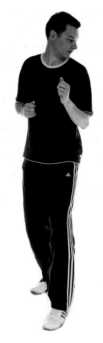

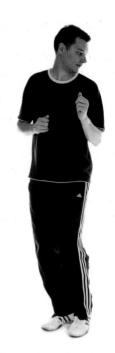

Step 4. Turn your head to look in the direction in which you wish to move next.

Step 5. Pull your front foot into your centre.

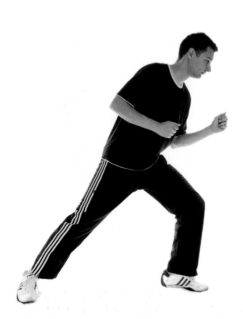

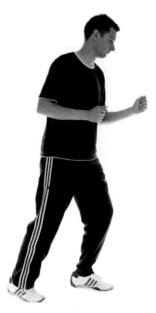

Step 6. Take a large step forward with your left leg.

Step 7. Lightly pull the back foot in so that you are standing in the same body position as in Step 1. Repeat as required.

## Pulling Back Foot and Stepping Backward

This is the second of three exercises that focuses on movement that includes a single step. A variation of the stepping forward movement is that of stepping backward, but instead of moving the leading leg first, you move the rear leg first. Stepping backward, then dragging your front foot in is a common method in which to make distance and also to change direction. When you move your feet across the ground, focus on sliding your foot lightly along the ground rather than lifting and stepping, so that both feet are in contact with the ground throughout the movement. Start slowly, building up speed as you become more comfortable with the movement. If you can remain on the balls of your feet throughout the exercise and keep light-footed, you should find that you can complete the movement more smoothly. You only have to lift your heel off the ground a small amount to be able to benefit from it. Practise this movement with either leg in the forward position.

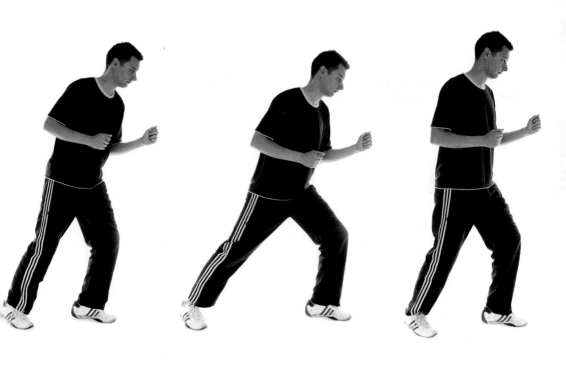

Step 1. Step forward with your left leg and stand in a relaxed fighting position.

Step 2. Take a large step backward with your right leg.

Step 3. Lightly pull the front foot in so that you are standing in the same body position as in Step 1. Repeat as required.

## Pulling Back Foot and Stepping Backward with Change of Direction

This is the final of three exercises that focuses on movement that includes a single step. The previous exercise is further developed here by adding a change of direction. In this exercise, you turn your head to look in the direction that you wish to move away from, then take your step backward away from that direction. When you move your feet across the ground, focus on sliding your foot lightly along the ground rather than lifting and stepping, so that both feet are in contact with the ground throughout the movement. Start slowly, building up as you become more comfortable with the movement. If you can remain on the balls of your feet throughout the exercise and keep light-footed, you should find that you can complete the movement more smoothly. You only have to lift your heel off the ground a tiny amount to be able to benefit. Practise this movement with either leg in the forward position.

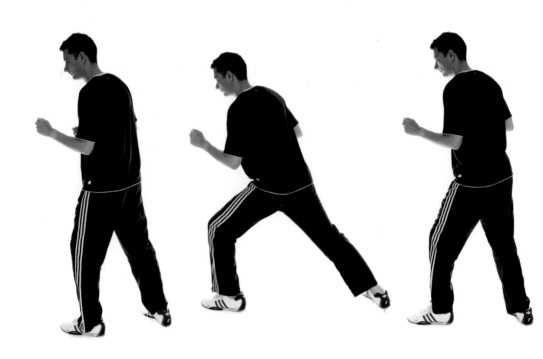

Step 1. Step forward with your left leg and stand in a relaxed fighting position.

Step 2. Take a large step backward with your right leg.

Step 3. Lightly pull the front foot in so that you are standing in the same body position as in Step 1.

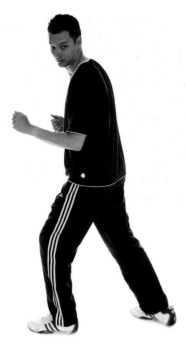

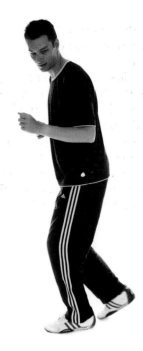

Step 4. Turn your head to look in the direction that you wish to move away from next.

Step 5. Pull your rear foot in towards your centre.

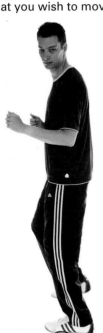

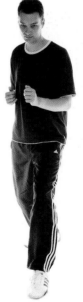

Step 6. Take a large step backward with your right leg.

Step 7. Lightly pull the front foot in so that you are standing in the same body position as in Step 1. Repeat as required, changing direction as you go.

## Moving Backward and Forward with a Split Step

A common move in many racket sports is footwork in order to movement forward, then change to moving backward. In fact, such movements are often tactically used in order to encourage an opponent to move into a more vulnerable position. Footwork training can enable you to be faster on your feet in order to make quick changes in direction.

This exercise makes use of a couple of different step types. You will be stepping backward, forward and using a technique called split step. Start by standing with your feet hip-width apart, then make a small jump that widens your base and bends your knees. This is the split step and it puts you in a position from which it is easy to move off. Take two steps forward, do a split step, then take two steps back. A good place to start would be to go forward three times and go back three times. If you keep a track of where you started, you should be able to check whether you make the same kind of distance going forward as you do when you are going backward.

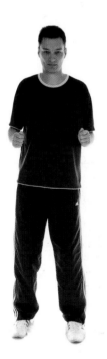
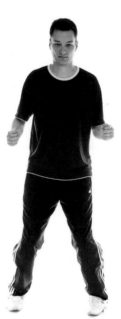
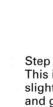
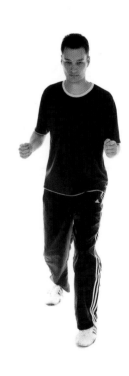

Step 1. Stand in a relaxed position with your feet one hip-width apart and firmly on the ground.

Step 2. Perform a split step. This is a small jump that slightly widens your base and gets your knees into a slightly bent position. You are now ready to move off.

Step 3. Take two steps forward.

Step 4. Perform a split step, as described in Step 2.

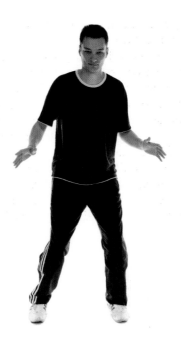

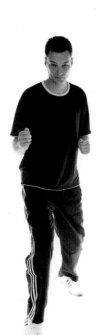

Step 5. Now take two steps back.

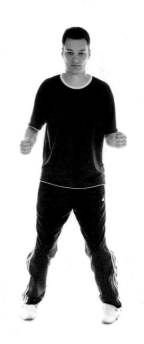

Step 6. Perform a split step, as described in Step 2. Repeat as required.

## Chassé and Side Step

Another common move in racket sports is that of moving side to side. One of the ways in which to practise this movement is by using a combination of chasséing and a side step. Start from your base and apply a split step, then move along to your side using a chasséing movement. After taking a couple of chassé steps, step across so that your back is facing forward. Then pull that foot back and chassé across to the other side, where you again take a step so that your back is facing forward. Step backward and chassé back to your starting position.

This exercise helps you to train in moving sideways using a couple of different step types and also to develop changing direction as you get to each side of the sequence. Practise this movement in both directions, so that you can move quickly both to your left and to your right and back again.

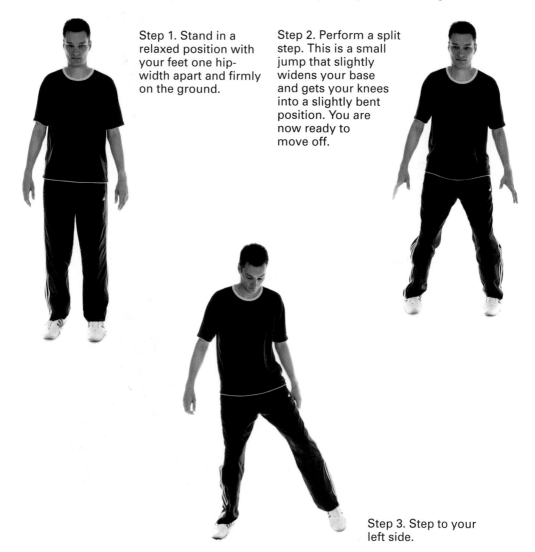

Step 1. Stand in a relaxed position with your feet one hip-width apart and firmly on the ground.

Step 2. Perform a split step. This is a small jump that slightly widens your base and gets your knees into a slightly bent position. You are now ready to move off.

Step 3. Step to your left side.

Step 4. Chassé to your left.
(A chassé is a triple-step pattern
with a gliding character using
a step-together-step
movement.)

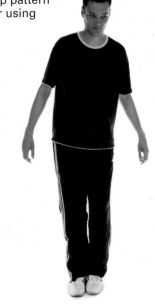

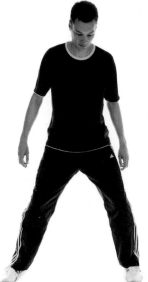

Step 5. Step to your left.

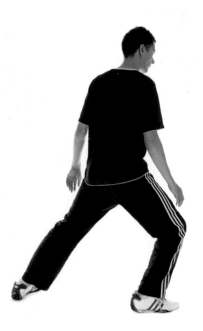

Step 6. Step across, so that your back is
facing to the front. Repeat on the other side.

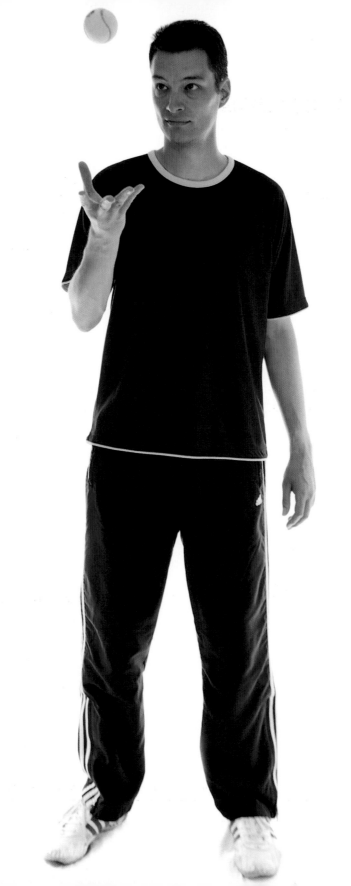

# 9 Co-ordination

*Coordination: the ability to move body parts in a specific sequence.*

**Co-ordination Exercises Summary**

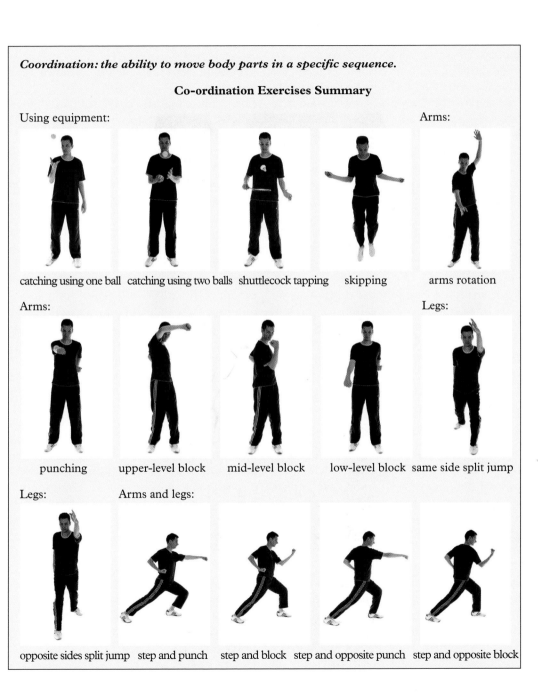

Using equipment:

Arms:

catching using one ball    catching using two balls    shuttlecock tapping    skipping    arms rotation

Arms:

Legs:

punching    upper-level block    mid-level block    low-level block    same side split jump

Legs:

Arms and legs:

opposite sides split jump    step and punch    step and block    step and opposite punch    step and opposite block

# ABOUT COORDINATION

Coordination refers to training for motor coordination of several limbs, or the coordination between various parts of the same movement or sequence to complete a prescribed motion. There are three main parts of the body involved in coordination, namely the muscles, the limbs and the nervous system. The purpose of developing coordination is to enable smooth and efficient movement. There are two main types of coordination:

• hand to eye coordination: this includes actions such as hitting or catching a moving target, for example in tennis, squash, cricket and baseball
• body coordination: this is the coordination of the limbs and the body, for example in gymnastics and the martial arts.

Coordination is one of those things that we start learning from a very young age through sheer repetitive trials. There is always scope to improve coordination and sport is an excellent way to make such training more enjoyable.

## BENEFITS OF TRAINING FOR COORDINATION

There are two main types of motor coordination. Firstly, gross motor skills include the general development of actions that utilize the large muscles. This includes actions such as running, jumping, bat and ball games, climbing and tumbling. Fine motor skills are those that enable the manipulation of small objects through the use of the hands. Tasks such as writing, drawing, typing and picking up objects all utilize fine motor skills. Developing gross motor skills is considered the foundation to learning fine motor skills. Take the example where babies first learn to move from the top downward. Very early on they develop their ability to move their arms

and hands. It is much later that they can pick up objects and pass them from one hand to another. The exercises in this chapter focus on the development of gross motor skills. Most sports require good coordination, for example:

• running: sprinting, long distance and hurdles
• ball games: football, basketball and rugby
• racket sports: tennis, badminton, squash and table tennis
• batting games: cricket, golf, baseball and hockey
• martial arts: karate, kung-fu, judo and aikido.

Training for coordination should result in smoother movement, better muscle control, improved body awareness and the improvement of trained actions, such as hitting and catching. It will also enable complicated movements with complex footwork to be completed more easily.

## IMPROVING COORDINATION

Repetition is the key to improving coordination. Such repeated efforts will train the muscles to behave in a certain way and be able to cope with complicated limb movement and combinations. Once a particular movement or combination has been mastered, it should feel effortless and second nature to complete that movement. Some training tips are listed below:

• start slow and then build up speed
• regularly perform repetitions
• go through the movement in your mind
• build up the complexity of the movement over time
• video your sequence or action so that you can review and monitor progress over time.

Further information on exercises that are beneficial for improving coordination can be found in Martin (2007) and Buschmann et al. (2001).

## SAFETY CONSIDERATIONS

Coordination training is likely to require a large clear area such as a hall or field. For exercises that include footwork, suitable footwear should be worn. Tiredness can reduce coordination in the short term, so ensure that suitable rest and recovery periods are incorporated into the workout. During training you should ensure:

- a safe training surface
- appropriate footwear and clothing
- suitable space for training
- awareness of your environment while moving.

If you are new to training for coordination, you may find that you lose balance or find it difficult to complete the movement. In this case, it is better to break down the movement into the steps that are described and perform them in a slow and controlled way.

## COORDINATION EXERCISES

### Catching Using One Ball

This is a simple exercise to improve hand to eye coordination. A tennis or juggling ball can be used. Here the focus is simply on catching the ball repeatedly using only one hand. To help control the ball, keep the throwing height to just above head height – any higher and you risk dropping the ball. Aim to keep the ball in the air under continuous movement for as long as possible. You could measure your progress over time by counting the number of times you can catch the ball before you drop it, or by counting how many catches you can do within a fixed amount of time.

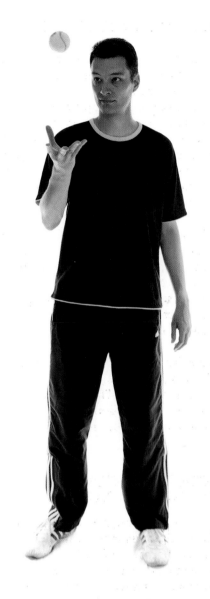

Throw the ball up so that it goes just above your head. Catch with the same hand. Repeat using the other hand.

**Catching Using Two Balls**

This exercise is similar to the previous exercise, but adds the complexity of using two balls and also using both hands in sequence. Again, you can use a tennis or juggling ball. Here the focus is on moving the balls in a circular motion and catching them alternately in each hand. To help control the ball, keep the throwing height to just above head height. Any higher and you risk dropping the balls. Aim to keep the balls in the air under continuous movement for as long as possible. You could measure your progress over time by counting the number of times you can complete a sequence before you drop the balls, or by counting how many sequences you can do within a fixed amount of time.

**Shuttlecock Tapping**

This exercise uses a racket to keep a shuttlecock up in the air for as long as possible. Here the focus is to control the action of the shuttlecock falling onto the racket head. This should help you to build an awareness of how far away the racket head is from your body and over time you should get better at being able to control the shuttle for an increasing number of hits. To help control the shuttlecock, keep the hitting height to just above head height. Aim to keep the shuttlecock in the air under continuous movement for as long as possible. You could measure your progress over time by counting the number of times you hit the shuttlecock before you drop it, or by counting how many contacts you can achieve within a fixed amount of time.

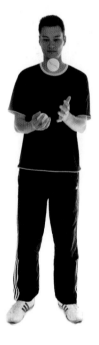

Throw one ball up so that it goes just above your head. At the same time, throw the other ball to the empty hand across your in front of your body. Catch the ball thrown up in the empty hand. Repeat as required. You should also try changing the direction of the ball-throwing.

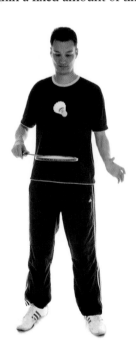

Hold a badminton racket in one hand and a shuttlecock in the other. Bounce the shuttlecock on the racket head, taking care that the shuttlecock does not fall to the ground.

## Skipping

This exercise works on improving overall body coordination. There are number of ways in which you can use a skipping rope for coordination exercises. This exercise it the simplest one and is a great place to start. Keep your feet together as you skip and work on improving the number of times you can jump over the rope before you trip and stop. Also aim gradually to increase the speed of your skipping. Once you are confident with this exercise, you could introduce different timings into your skipping, or even introduce a running skip action, by alternating your feet as they go over the skipping rope.

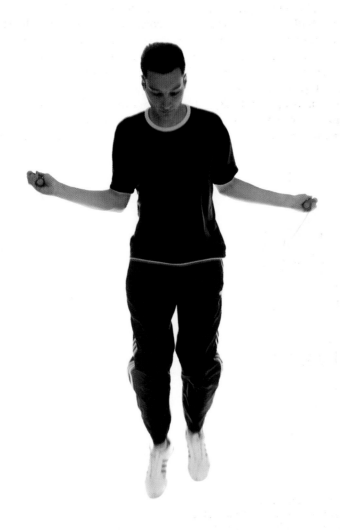

Skip, with both feet jumping over the rope at the same time.

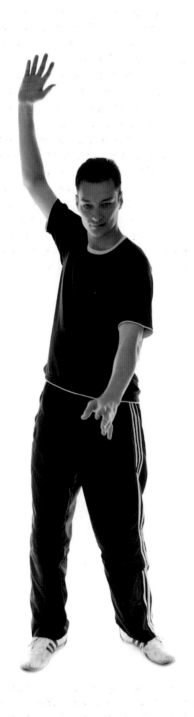

## Arms Rotation

This is an exercise that is beneficial for developing arm coordination. Stand in a comfortable position and rotate both of your arms in an opposite direction from each other. This exercise may look simple, but at first you are likely to need to concentrate in order to get your arms to rotate in opposite directions. Done properly, this exercise can use the full range of motion of your arms and therefore can be a good exercise for maintaining flexibility in your arms. Once you are comfortable performing this exercise, reverse direction on both sides.

Rotate both arms in opposite directions. Try to use the full range of motion of your arms. Once you get comfortable performing this exercise, reverse the direction of movement of the arms.

## Punching

This exercise is taken from karate. Martial arts such as karate can be excellent for developing coordination. They require high degrees of coordination between the arms, legs and head. Training includes the learning of complex sequences of movement called katas and consists of numerous repetitions to achieve smooth body coordination. It is through the thousands of repetitions of each movement that such complex techniques and sequences can become second nature, looking smooth and effortless when performed.

This punching exercise focuses on upper body coordination and is one that is often taught to beginners in karate. You start by holding out a punch on one side of the body, then as you retract that arm you punch out with the other side. There is great deal of technique involved in learning how to punch. However, for the purpose of this exercise you should focus on the coordination required to push one arm out and at the same time retract the other. You should finish the movement on both arms at the same time and they should move roughly at the same speed. When you first try this exercise you might find that you can only move one arm at a time, but with practice you should be able to get both of your arms to complete different actions at the same time. Do not let your elbows stick out during the movement. They should remain in line with the rest of your arm at all times.

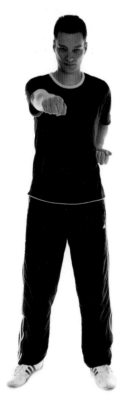

Step 1. Stand with one arm stretched out in front of you and the other fist just above your hips. Both hands should be closed.

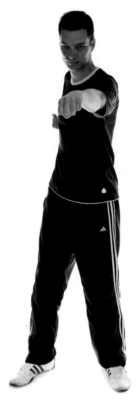

Step 2. Bring the outstretched arm back to just above your hip and push forward the other arm simultaneously. Repeat as required.

**Upper-Level Block**

A range of techniques that are taught very early on in karate are blocks, which require mostly upper body coordination. These exercises are selected from those that look deceptively easy when performed by an expert, yet beginners struggle with the coordination until they have completed a number of training sessions. This is the first block of three and is used for blocking upper body attacks in karate. Here it is presented for its use as an upper body coordination exercise. As with the punching exercise, this one requires each arm to perform a different action at the same time and to complete those actions simultaneously and using the same kind of speed. It is for this reason that it can be difficult.

Start by preparing your arms for the block. One arm is raised in front of you and the other fist rests just above your hip. Slightly lower the raised arm and lift up the other arms so that your forearms are crossed in front of you. Both of your arms should then continue the movement through so that the opposite arm finishes raised and the previously raised arm now rests by your side.

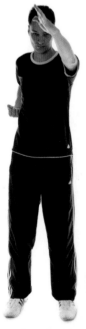 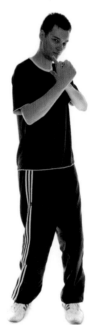 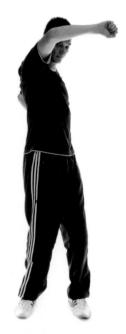

Step 1. Stand with one arm stretched out in front of you as shown and the other fist just above your hips. The raised hand should be open.

Step 2. Bring the outstretched arm back to just above your hip and push forward the other arm simultaneously. Both arms should cross in front of your face.

Step 3. Follow the movement through, with the lifting arm ending up raised with the palm turned away from you. The other arm should be by your side, with the fist resting just above your hip. Note that the position of the raised arm is such that it should block an upper level attack. Repeat as required.

## Mid-Level Block

This is another block that is taught early on in karate. This exercise also requires mostly upper body coordination. It looks deceptively easy when performed by an expert, but beginners struggle with the coordination until they have completed a number of training sessions. This is the second block of three and is used for blocking mid-level attacks in karate. Here it is presented for its use as an upper body coordination exercise. As with the previous punching and blocking exercise, this one requires each arm to perform a different action at the same time and to complete those actions simultaneously and using the same kind of speed. It can therefore be difficult.

Start by preparing your arms for the block. One arm is outstretched in front of you and the other arm is raised by the side of your head with the palm side of the fist facing outwards. The raised arm should be bent at the elbow and the knuckles should face outwards. You then pull the outstretched arm back to just above your hip and push the raised arm in a circular motion to resting in front of you. Add a forearm rotation to this arm so that the palm of the fist faces towards you at the end.

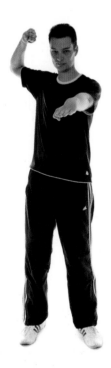

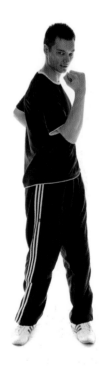

Step 1. Stand with one arm stretched out in front of you as shown and the other arm raised by the side of your head with the palm side of the fist facing outwards. The raised arm should be bent at the elbow.

Step 2. Bring the outstretched arm back to just above your hip and push forward the other arm simultaneously. Repeat as required.

## Low-Level Block

This is another block that is taught early on in karate. This exercise also requires mostly upper body coordination and can look deceptively simple. This is the final block of three and is used for blocking low-level attacks in karate. Here it is presented for its use as an upper body coordination exercise. As with the previous punching and blocking exercises, this one requires each arm to perform a different action at the same time and to complete those actions simultaneously and using the same

kind of speed. It can therefore be difficult.

Start by preparing your arms for the block. One arm is outstretched in front of you and the other arm is raised by the side of your head with the palm side of the fist facing inwards. The raised fist should be near your ear and the elbows of both of arms should be close. You then pull the outstretched arm back to just above your hip and push the raised arm downward in front of you. Add a forearm rotation to this arm so that the palm of the fist faces downward at the end.

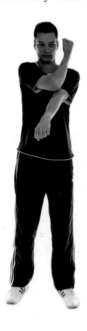
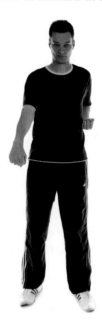

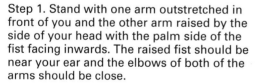

Step 1. Stand with one arm outstretched in front of you and the other arm raised by the side of your head with the palm side of the fist facing inwards. The raised fist should be near your ear and the elbows of both of the arms should be close.

Step 2. Pull the outstretched arm back to just above your hip and push the raised arm downward in front of you. Add a forearm rotation to this arm so that the palm of the fist faces downward at the end. Repeat as required.

## Same Side Split Jump

This is a simple exercise that is often used for warm-ups, as it can provide a quick cardiovascular workout if sufficient repetitions are performed quickly. Here it is presented for developing upper and lower body coordina-

tion. Start with the arm and leg of the same side out in front of you, then jump so that the other arm and leg are in front of you. Continue to perform this jumping action, trying to go faster and faster while also maintaining the coordination of the movement.

Step 1. Stand in a relaxed position with your feet one hip-width apart and firmly on the ground. Then split jump, so that your left arm and left leg move forward and your right arm and right leg move backward at the same time.

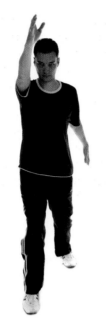

Step 2. Alternate and repeat as required.

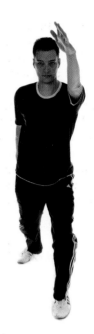

**Opposite Sides Split Jump**

This is another simple exercise that is often used for warm-ups, as it can provide a quick cardiovascular workout if sufficient repetitions are performed quickly. Here it is presented for developing upper and lower body coordination and it builds on the previous one by adding the complexity of using opposing arms and legs in sequence. This exercise is often found to be far more difficult to coordinate than the previous one. Start with the arm and leg of opposite sides out in front of you, then jump so that the other arm and leg are then in front of you. Continue to perform this jumping action, trying to go faster and faster while also maintaining the coordination of the movement.

Step 1. Stand in a relaxed position with your feet one hip-width apart and firmly on the ground. Then split jump, so that your left arm and right leg move forward and your right arm and left leg move backward at the same time.

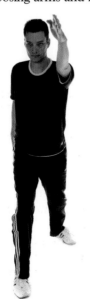

Step 2. Alternate and repeat as required.

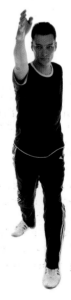

## Step and Punch

This exercise builds on the punching exercise described earlier in this chapter. Here, movement with the legs is added so that you perform a stepping punch as you would do in karate training. The challenge is to keep the motion of the legs and the arms in sequence, so that the movement of the arms and the legs finishes at the same time.

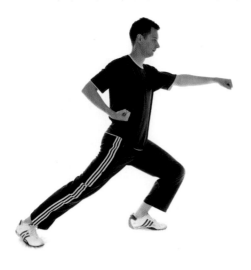

Step 1. Stand in a relaxed position with your feet one hip-width apart and firmly on the ground. Push your left leg forward. Slide your foot lightly along the ground. End with your front knee bent. Also, ready your arms so that they are in the position as described in the 'Punching' exercise. The same arm and leg should be in front.

Step 2. Prepare for the next punch by sliding your right foot towards your centre.

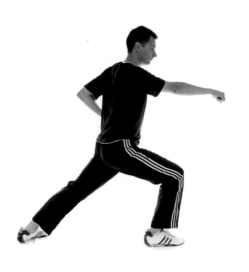

Step 3. Step through, so that you are standing with your right leg in front and the right knee bent. Simultaneously, exchange the hands with your foot movement, such that you complete a stepping punch. Repeat as required.

## Step and Block

This exercise, like the previous one, focuses on developing the coordination between the arms and legs. Here, movement is added to the mid-level block that was described earlier in this chapter. The challenge is to keep the motion of the legs and the arms in sequence, so that the movement of the arms and the legs finishes at the same time. The exercise is described below using the mid-level block, but any of the blocks presented in this chapter can be used with this footwork.

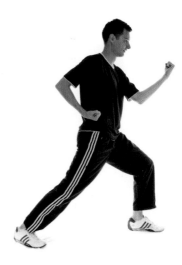

Step 1. Stand in a relaxed position with your feet one hip-width apart and firmly on the ground. Push your left leg forward. Slide your foot lightly along the ground. End with your front knee bent. Also, ready your arms so that they are in the position as described in the 'Mid-Level Block' exercise. The same arm and leg should be in front.

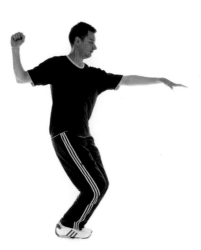

Step 2. Prepare for the next block by sliding your right foot towards your centre.

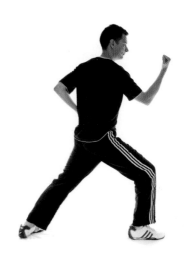

Step 3. Step through, so that you are standing with your right leg in front and the right knee bent. Simultaneously, exchange the hands with your foot movement, such that you complete a stepping block. Repeat as required.

## Step and Opposite Punch

This exercise builds on the step and punch exercise described earlier in this chapter. This time, you should punch with the opposite arm to the leg that is in front. The chal-lenge is to keep the motion of the legs and the arms in sequence, so that the movement of the arms and the legs finishes at the same time. This time each limb will be performing a more unique action than before.

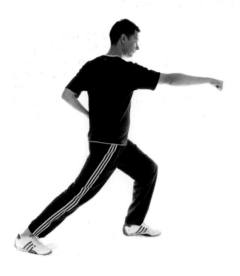

Step 1. Stand in a relaxed position with your feet one hip-width apart and firmly on the ground. Push your left leg forward. Slide your foot lightly along the ground. End with your front knee bent. Also, ready your arms so that they are in the position as described in the 'Punching' exercise. The opposite arm and leg should be in front.

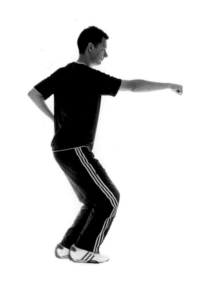

Step 2. Prepare for the next punch by sliding your right foot towards your centre.

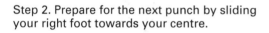

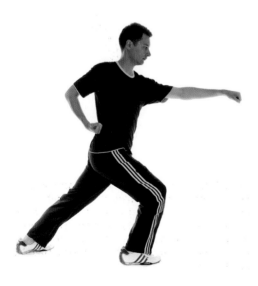

Step 3. Slide your right foot towards your centre and then step through, so that you are standing with your right leg in front and the right knee bent. Simultaneously, exchange the hands with your foot movement, such that you complete a stepping punch. Repeat as required.

## Step and Opposite Block

This exercise, like the previous one, focuses on developing the coordination of the arms and legs. This time, the aim is to block with the opposite arm to the leg that is in front. The challenge is to keep the motion of the legs and the arms in sequence, so that the movement of the arms and legs finishes at the same time. The exercise is described below using the mid-level block, but any of the blocks presented in this chapter can be used in this sequence.

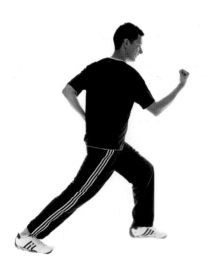

Step 1. Stand in a relaxed position with your feet one hip-width apart and firmly on the ground. Push your left leg forward. Slide your foot lightly along the ground. End with your front knee bent. Also, ready your arms so that they are in the position as described in the 'Mid-Level Block' exercise. The opposite arm and leg should be in front.

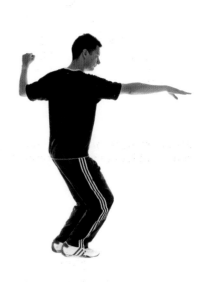

Step 2. Prepare for the next block by sliding your right foot towards your centre.

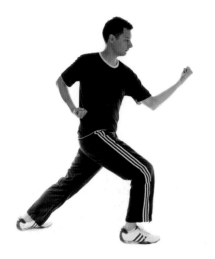

Step 3. Slide your right foot towards your centre and then step through, so that you are standing with your right leg in front and the right knee bent. Simultaneously, exchange the hands with your foot movement, such that you complete a stepping block. Repeat as required.

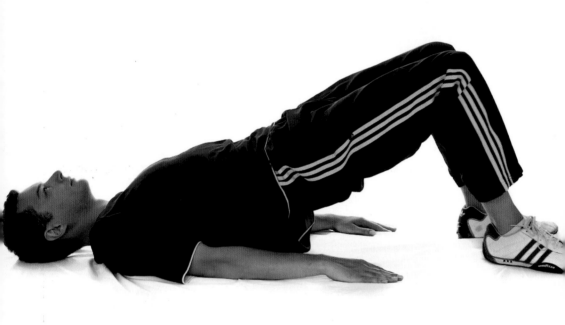

# 10  Posture

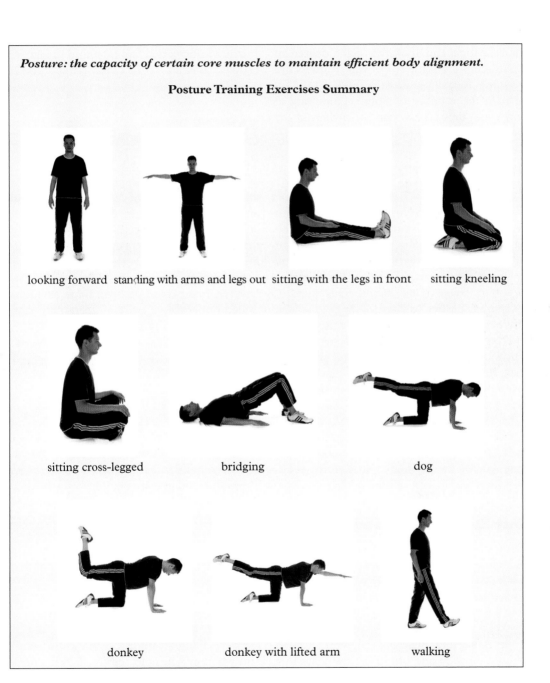

*Posture: the capacity of certain core muscles to maintain efficient body alignment.*

**Posture Training Exercises Summary**

looking forward   standing with arms and legs out   sitting with the legs in front   sitting kneeling

sitting cross-legged          bridging                    dog

donkey        donkey with lifted arm          walking

# ABOUT POSTURE

In normal healthy muscles, there will always be a few muscle fibres contracting at any one time, even during sleep. This action gives normal posture to the body. This is called muscle tone and it is the slight degree of contraction by some fibres whilst others are relaxing. Relaxation is when there is a reduction in the number of fibres contracting at any one time. This can be achieved by conscious effort and assisted relaxation.

# BENEFITS OF TRAINING FOR POSTURE

Training to improve your posture is all about increasing awareness of your body position and also trying to train yourself to keep good posture naturally, without having to think about it. This comes down to teaching the body to create good habits. This kind of exercise is particularly useful for people who are out of shape. Good posture can give you the competitive edge in many sports and is key in sports like golf, martial arts and baseball. Bad habits can result in bad posture, for example not sitting up straight, slouching when standing and looking at the ground when walking. Uneven movement can also result in bad posture, since some muscles will stretch more than others and create imbalances in the body. Such imbalances can increase the risk of injury.

# IMPROVING POSTURE

Poor posture can result from bad habits, therefore improving posture can take time. Your head should be level so that you can look directly ahead of you without feeling any tension in the neck and shoulders. Many postural exercises focus on developing control over the muscles in the body, so you should move in and out of the exercises in a smooth and controlled manner. In this way, if you feel any jerkiness in your movement, it will indicate where you need to work on developing your muscle control. Pilates and yoga are good examples of activities that focus on posture and muscle control. Further information can be found in Martin (2009), Bussell (2005), Lawrence (2007) and Robinson et al. (2002).

# SAFETY CONSIDERATIONS

There should be no discomfort felt during any of the exercises for training posture. As with any activity, do not continue if you feel any pain or clicking in the joints. Do not attempt these exercises when you are fatigued. If you have any current back or muscular injuries, seek medical advice before trying any of the exercises in this chapter. It is best to perform these exercises under supervision so that technique and alignment can be checked.

# POSTURE EXERCISES

### Looking Forward
This is a simple exercise for developing awareness of how you stand and whether you hold tension in your neck and shoulders. Stand with your feet hip-width apart, then focus on relaxing your shoulders so that they drop. Look directly ahead and be aware of how you would normally hold your gaze when you are moving around or standing. Think about how straight your back is. You want to be upright whilst also maintaining the natural curvature of your back.

### Standing with Arms and Legs Out
Similar to the previous exercise, this one is for developing awareness of how you stand and whether you hold tension in your neck

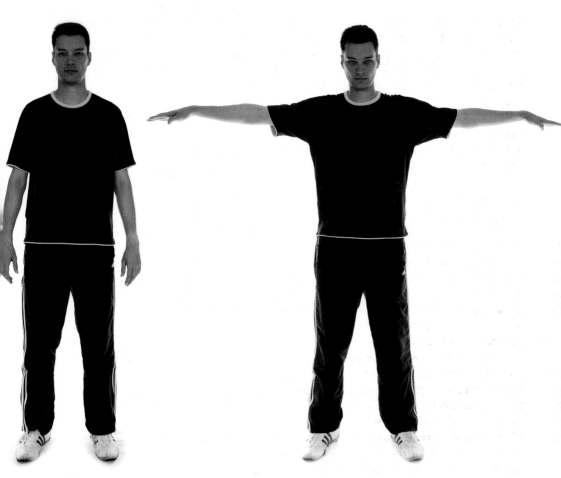

Stand with your back against a wall and look straight ahead. Ensure that your head and back are resting on the wall. Your back should maintain the natural curve of the spine and should not be forced into a straight shape. Repeat as required.

Stand comfortably with your feet hip-width apart and firmly on the ground. Your back should maintain the natural curve of the spine and should not be forced into a straight shape. Keep the arms parallel to the ground and in line with your shoulders. Repeat as required.

and shoulders. Stand with your feet hip-width apart, then focus on relaxing your shoulders so that they drop. Look directly ahead and be aware of how you would normally hold your gaze when you are moving around or standing. Think about how straight your back is. You want to be

upright whilst also maintaining the natural curvature of your back. Then lift your arms out to your side until they are in line with your shoulders. It is better to perform this exercise in front of a mirror so that you can check your arms are in line and are at the same height.

## Sitting with Legs in Front

The most basic sitting position is with your legs stretched out straight in front of you. This simple exercise helps to raise awareness of how you sit and your overall posture. Many yoga poses use this as a starting position, then work on moving the rest of the body into the correct position. Make sure that your back is straight and your knees are not bent. Do not let your hands rest on the floor behind you. Instead, place the hands lightly on your legs or in front of you. This will help to ensure that you keep your back straight and upright and remain balanced.

Varying the position of the feet will vary the muscles that are engaged during this stretch. For example, if you pull your feet back, you will engage the hamstrings and the calves. If you point the feet, you will feel the muscles on the front of the legs working. The further apart you push your feet, the more you will engage the hip adductors. Do not hold any tension in your neck or shoulders and keep your gaze forward.

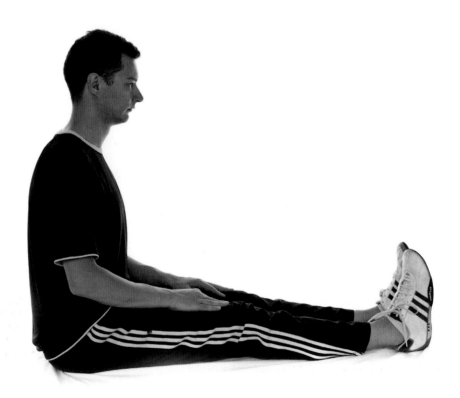

Sit with both of your legs straight out in front of you and your knees, heels and big toes touching. Push the back of your knees into the ground and do not let your legs rotate outwards. Place your palms flat on your lap with your fingers pointing forward. Keep your back straight and your shoulders down and pushed back slightly so that your chest is opened up. Push your pelvis slightly forward and bring your navel in slightly towards your spine. Hold your gaze parallel to the floor. Do not hold any tension in your neck or shoulders.

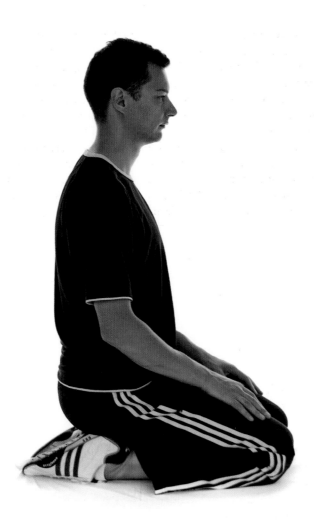

Kneel with your feet either side of you, your hands resting lightly on the knees and your bottom touching the ground between your feet. The tops of your feet should be in contact with the ground and your toes should be pointing backward. Your thighs should be parallel. Keep your back straight and your shoulders down and pushed back slightly so that your chest is opened up. Push your pelvis slightly forward. Hold your gaze parallel to the floor. Do not hold any tension in your neck or shoulders.

### Sitting Kneeling

This is an example of a position that looks simple, yet can be very challenging. In this basic kneeling position, your back is straight and your bottom is resting firmly on your feet. Do not rest your hands on the ground behind you. It is best to rest them lightly on the knees. This exercise works your quadriceps and your knee and ankle joints. You may feel stiff around the joints when you come out of this position. In which case, flexing the knees and rotating the ankles can be beneficial. Do not hold any tension in your neck or shoulders and keep your gaze forward.

## Sitting Cross-Legged

Some find sitting on the ground cross-legged difficult, while for others it is effortless. The aim is to be able to sit in this position for extended amounts of time. You should have your back straight and your bottom resting firmly on the ground. Do not rest your hands on the ground behind you. It is best to rest them lightly on your knees. This exercise works your knee and ankle joints, so you may feel stiff around the joints when you come out of this position. In which case, flexing the knees and rotating the ankles can be beneficial. Do not hold any tension in your neck or shoulders and keep your gaze forward.

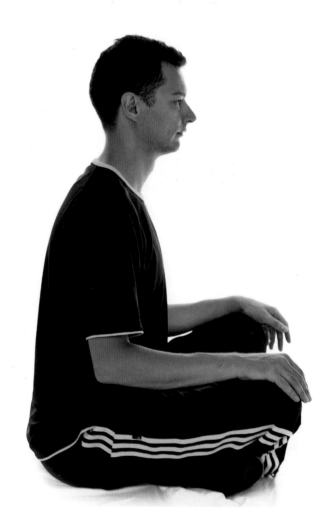

Sit on the ground cross-legged with your feet firmly under you and your hands resting lightly on the knees. Keep your back straight and your shoulders down and pushed back slightly so that your chest is opened up. Push your pelvis slightly forward. Hold your gaze parallel to the floor. Do not hold any tension in your neck or shoulders.

## Bridging

This exercise is good for developing the muscles along the spine. Start on the ground with your knees bent. Slowly lift your back off the ground until your hips are in line with your knees. You should have the feeling of lifting each vertebra one at a time. Also, the action should be smooth and continuous as you move from one vertebra to the next. Wherever you feel a jerkiness in your movement, that will indicate where you need to focus on improving control over those muscles. Similarly, you must employ the same control going back down into the starting position. This exercise must be completed slowly. You could engage the pelvic floor muscles while doing this exercise.

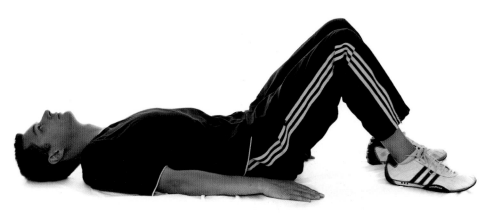

Step 1. Lie on your back with knees bent and feet flat on the ground. Your arms should rest by your sides.

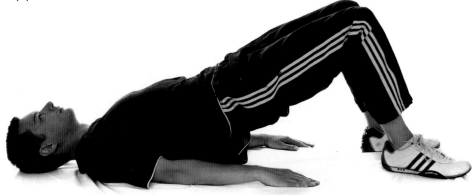

Step 2. Lift the hips off the ground, then roll each vertebra one at a time until your hips are in line with your knees. Slowly curl back down again. Repeat as required.

## Donkey

This exercise is good for working the core muscles and the gluteals. Start on the ground on all fours, then slowly lift one leg off the ground until it is in line with your back. You should look towards the ground throughout this exercise. You then replace that leg back on the ground and perform the exercise on the other side. The movement must be completed slowly. You could engage the pelvic floor muscles while doing this exercise.

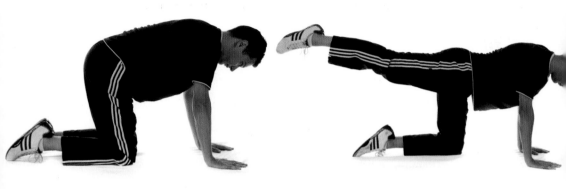

Step 1. Start on the ground on all fours. You should look at the ground throughout this movement.

Step 2. Stretch one leg straight behind you in a slow and controlled manner. It should be in line with your back at the end of the movement. Return to Step 1 and perform the exercise with the other leg. Repeat as required.

## Dog

This exercise is also good for working the core muscles and the gluteals. Start on the ground on all fours, then slowly lift one leg off the ground. However, this time you must keep it bent at 90 degrees throughout the movement. Stop when the thigh of your raised leg is in line with your back. You should look towards the ground throughout this exercise. You then replace that leg back on the ground and perform the exercise on the other side. The movement must be completed slowly. You could engage the pelvic floor muscles while doing this exercise.

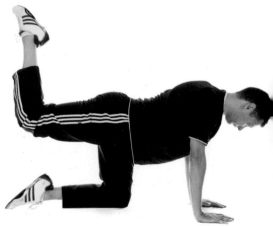

Start on the ground on all fours, then slowly lift one leg off the ground, keeping it bent at 90 degrees throughout the movement. Stop when the thigh of your raised leg is in line with your back. You should look towards the ground throughout this exercise.

## Donkey with Lifted Arm

This exercise is good for working the whole of the abdominals. Start on the ground on all fours, as you did for the previous donkey exercise. Slowly lift one leg off the ground until it is in line with your back. At the same time, lift the opposite arm out in front so that it is also in line with your back at the end of the movement. Look towards the ground throughout this exercise. You then replace that leg and arm back on the ground and perform the exercise on the other side. The movement must be completed slowly. You could engage the pelvic floor muscles while doing this exercise.

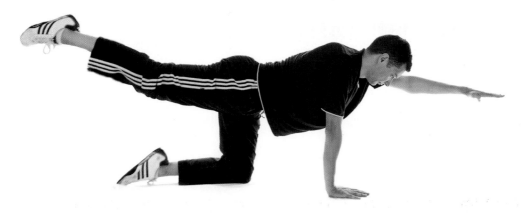

Start on the ground on all fours. You should look at the ground throughout this movement. Stretch one leg straight behind you and the opposite arm out in front of you in a slow and controlled manner. They should be in line with your back at the end of the movement. Return them to the ground and repeat with the other arm and leg. Repeat as required.

## Walking

The final exercise in this chapter focuses on using good posture when walking. Using good posture when walking should help you to feel more confident, as well as reducing the risk of back pain. You should not arch your back when you walk or lean forward or backward. Keep your gaze as parallel to the ground as possible. Do not be tempted always to look at the ground when walking. Open up your chest and let your neck and shoulders relax. This will also help to keep your back in proper alignment. Do not push your head forward.

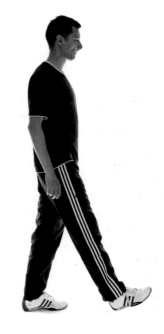

You should always try to be aware of your posture during walking and bear in mind the good posture walking tips.

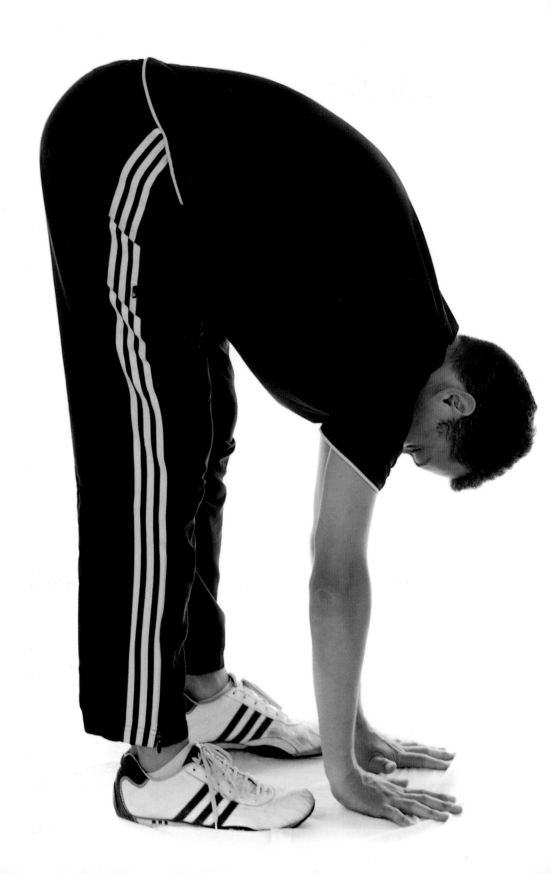

# 11    Flexibility

*Flexibility: the range of movement around a joint or the amount of resistance to movement.*

## Flexibility Exercises Summary

Arms:                                                              Legs:

| arm lifts in front | arm lifts to the side | triceps stretch | calves stretch |

Legs:

| standing hip adductors | sitting hip adductors | hamstring stretch | standing quadriceps |

Legs:                                                              Back:

| lying quadriceps stretch | gluteals stretch | leaning backward | waist twist |

## ABOUT FLEXIBILITY

Flexibility is the range of movement around a joint or the amount of resistance to movement. Flexibility training normally takes the form of stretching. In general, flexibility reduces with age and a lack of taking the body through movements that utilize its full range. It often goes unnoticed, as the reason inflexibility occurs is due to not moving in a particular way. Therefore, you are far more likely to notice any changes in your flexibility when you try doing something that is not a part of your normal routine, like taking up a new activity. As flexibility decreases, the range of muscle movement becomes shorter and the muscles become tighter. This increases the risk of injury, particularly when taking part in any form of sport or activity. Flexibility training requires a consistent and regular approach. In fact, if you are not used to stretching, you are likely to feel muscles soreness once you start to train. This alone is enough to put the majority off incorporating any type of stretching into their training.

There are a number of different ways of stretching. However, the exercises in this chapter focus on static stretching. This is where the body is moved into a particular position in a slow and controlled motion. The position is then held for a short time and the muscles allowed to relax into the stretch. The exercise can be repeated after a short pause. Once you are able to hold the position for increasing amounts of time, you may find that you can gradually go a little bit further. Eventually you will come to the limit of your flexibility range. It is this limit that you will be looking to develop through flexibility training.

## BENEFITS OF TRAINING FOR FLEXIBILITY

Training for flexibility is an excellent complement to any other type of training activity. The exercises can easily be incorporated into the cool-down section of any workout. Also, because the exercises presented here are static, it is possible to practise some of these while doing other things, for example while watching television or lying down. Training for flexibility will help to:

• reduce the risk of injury
• improve suppleness
• delay the effects of aging.

Like other training, the body should be given appropriate rest and recovery periods between workouts, although simple stretches could be incorporated into your daily routine.

## IMPROVING FLEXIBILITY

Flexibility programmes are best arranged around individual requirements. Each person will have a specific history, or imbalances in the body caused by socio-environmental factors. They will also have peculiarities in terms of their medical history that should be taken into account. For this reason, it is advised that any flexibility training is done under suitable supervision.

Flexibility training is a core part of certain sports and activities, for example:

• yoga
• gymnastics
• dancing
• martial arts.

Since flexibility training can be hard work, it can be more effective to train in a group environment. Taking part in an activity that incorporates stretching into the training should make it more enjoyable and satisfying. Further information can be found in Martin (2009), Brown (2003), Norris (2001) and Iyengar (1991).

The key to improving flexibility is to not expect too much too quickly. It is likely to take several training sessions before any improvements become apparent. While performing the exercises, it is important to not go too far. Stop as soon as you feel any pain. Some amount of muscle soreness is to be expected, however. You should ensure that you incorporate appropriate rest periods into your training programme so that your muscles have a chance to recover between workouts. The exercises in this chapter are described using a step-by-step approach. One method you could use to keep track of your progress is by keeping a note of when you are able to complete each successive step of an exercise. You could also keep notes on how you feel when doing the exercises. In this way, you will be able to monitor your progress. Once you have mastered these exercises, you should find them effortless.

When starting training for flexibility, you may find that you can perform some exercises better than others, or even that you are more flexible in certain muscles than others. It is important to develop your flexibility in a holistic way, so that you smooth out any differences in flexibility, for example from one side of the body to the other.

## SAFETY CONSIDERATIONS

You should not train on an empty stomach or immediately after a heavy meal. Your breathing should be comfortable during the exercises; if you start to have trouble breathing, stop immediately. Pay attention to any safety instructions. Also, remember that it is better to practise an easier step for longer than to struggle with a more difficult step before you are ready. If you are uncomfortable with any exercise, do not attempt it.

## FLEXIBILITY EXERCISES

### Arm Lifts in Front

This exercise focuses on the muscles in the arms and utilizing as much of the range of motion as possible. Start in a kneeling position with your arms resting by your sides. Raise your arms in front of you and continue

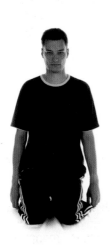

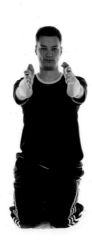

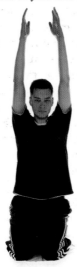

Step 1. Start in a kneeling position on the ground. Rest your arms by your side. Push your pelvis slightly forward, open up the chest and gaze forward.

Step 2. Raise your arms in front of you, keeping them straight the whole time.

Step 3. Continue to lift your arms as high as they will go. Repeat as required.

to lift them as high above your head as possible. Your arms should remain straight throughout this exercise. While you are seated in the kneeling position, remember to open up your chest and keep your gaze forward. Tilting your pelvis slightly forward will help to keep your back upright.

## Arm Lifts to the Side

This exercise also focuses on the muscles in the arms and utilizing as much of the range of motion as possible. However, this time you will be lifting your arms round the sides of your body instead of in front. Start in a kneeling position with your arms resting by your sides. Raise your arms to your sides and continue to lift them as high above your head as possible. Your arms should remain straight throughout this exercise. While you are seated in the kneeling position, remember to open up your chest and keep your gaze forward. Tilting your pelvis slightly forward will help to keep your back upright.

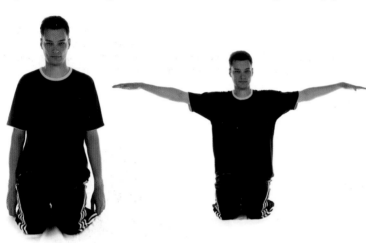

Step 1. Start in a kneeling position on the ground. Rest your arms by your side. Push your pelvis slightly forward, open up the chest and gaze forward.

Step 2. Raise your arms to your sides, keeping them straight the whole time.

Step 3. Continue to lift your arms as high as they will go. Repeat as required.

## Triceps Stretch

This exercise focuses on stretching the triceps. Start in a kneeling position with your arms resting by your sides. Raise one arm behind your head and hold the elbow with the other hand. You should not place any pressure on your neck or lean forward with your head. While you are seated in the kneeling position, remember to tilt your pelvis slightly forward, as this will help to keep your back upright. The exercise is shown using both a front view and a rear view.

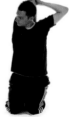

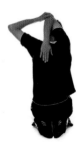

Start in a kneeling position with your arms resting by your sides. Raise one arm behind your head and hold the elbow with the other hand.

Rear view of the triceps stretch.

## Calves Stretch

This exercise focuses on stretching the calf muscles. This is a simple exercise that can be easily incorporated into the cool-down part of a workout. Many people involved in running use this exercise at the end of their workout. Start by standing near a wall and then, with one leg forward, lean on the wall. This should produce a stretch in the calf of your rear leg. You should then repeat on the other leg.

## Standing Hip Adductors Stretch

The exercise focuses on developing the hip adductor muscles. This exercise is an important one if you are trying to work towards doing the splits. These muscles are generally very tight since they are normally rarely used. For this reason, you should take extra care when trying this exercise as you do not want to overstretch. Stand with your legs as far apart as possible and try to relax the body into the stretch. You must ensure that your legs are not so wide apart that you slip or feel uncomfortable. You are aiming to stretch your legs as far apart as possible over time. If you can reach, then you should rest your palms flat on the ground. Your legs must remain straight throughout the exercise and you are likely to feel soreness around the knees when holding this position.

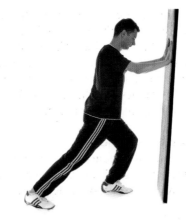

Stand two feet away from a wall, then move one leg forward and lean on the wall. Ensure that both of your heels are firmly on the ground. The stretch should be felt in your rear leg.

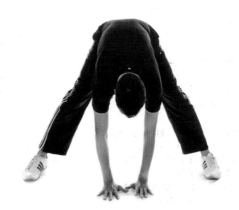

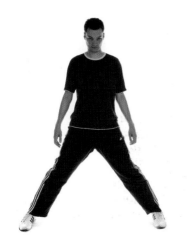

LEFT: Step 1. Stand with your feet as far apart as is comfortable. Your feet should point forward.

ABOVE: Step 2. If you can reach, support your weight by placing your hands down on the ground in front of you. Keep the legs straight. Repeat as required.

## Sitting Hip Adductors Stretch

If you are worried about slipping in the previous exercise, you could try this one instead. This exercise also focuses on developing the hip adductor muscles. It is also an important one if you are trying to work towards doing the splits. These muscles are generally very tight since they are normally rarely used, so care should be taken not to overstretch. Sit with your feet together and try to relax the body into the stretch. You are aiming to get your knees as close as possible to the ground over time. If you can already get your knees onto the ground, you could try placing your palms on the ground in front of you and pushing them forward.

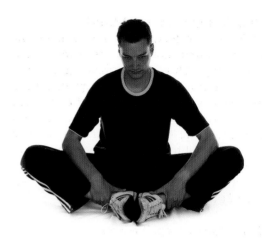

Sit with the feet together on the ground and push the knees down using your elbows.

## Hamstring Stretch

This exercise focuses on developing the hamstring muscles. It is another exercise that can be easily incorporated into the cool-down part of a workout. The hamstrings are the major muscle group in the back of the legs. This stretch utilizes them by using the forward bending action to achieve the required position. You are aiming to reach as far forward as possible, so that you are able to place your palms on to the ground. You are likely to also feel a stretch along your back. If you are not able to reach the ground, you should just hang forward. Do not bounce or bend the knees in order to reach the ground. You need to let the muscles have time to develop in order to reach the ground safely. Do not perform this exercise if you feel dizzy at all.

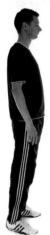
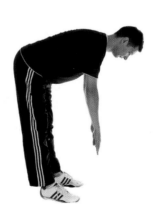
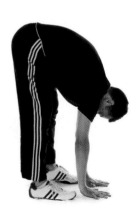

Step 1. Stand with your feet one hip-width apart. Allow your upper body to relax and keep the legs straight.

Step 2. Slowly bend forward from the hips. Your legs must remain straight at all times.

Step 3. If you can reach, then support your weight by placing your palms onto the ground and hold. Repeat.

## Standing Quadriceps Stretch

This exercise focuses on the development of the muscle group in the front of the upper legs. This simple standing exercise for achieving a stretch in the quadriceps is easily incorporated into the cool-down part of a workout. Start in a standing position and bend one of your knees so that your foot is raised towards your bottom. If you are able to reach, you should use both of your hands to hold your foot in position. Do not lean forward.

## Lying Quadriceps Stretch

If you have space, you could try the lying down version of the previous exercise. You lie on your front and bend the knees. You could try both legs at the same time, using your hands to hold the feet in order to bring them safely in closer to your bottom. The standing version is useful because you can easily perform this exercise outdoors, or on other surfaces that are unsuitable for lying down.

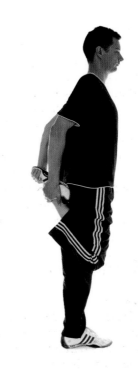

Bend one of your knees and bring the foot of that leg as close as possible to your bottom and hold. You may use your hands to support the raised foot. Try to keep the knees together. Repeat this exercise on the other leg.

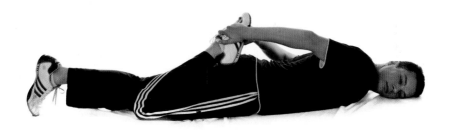

Lie on the ground face down. Bend one of your knees and bring the foot as close as possible to your bottom and hold. You may use your hands to support the raised foot.

## Gluteals Stretch

This exercise focuses on developing the muscles in the gluteals and deep muscles in the leg. You lie on your back and bend your knees, then rest one of your ankles on the other knee. Once in this position, raise the supporting leg off the ground while using one hand to bring that leg closer to the body. Use the other hand to push lightly on the knee of the leg in front. If you are very tight in these muscles, you will find that you won't be able to bring the knee very close to your chest. As you improve, you should notice that you are able to bring the knee in closer over time.

Step 1. Lay on your back on the ground and bend both of the knees, keeping the feet flat on the ground. Rest your arms by your side.

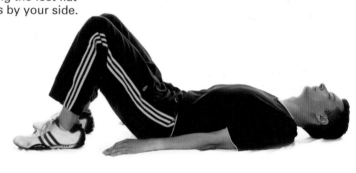

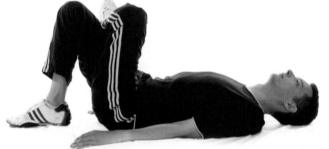

Step 2. Raise one leg and rest that foot on the opposite knee.

Step 3. Use one hand to hold the supporting leg and pull towards your chest. You are aiming to get the knee as close to your chest as possible. With the other hand, you should lightly push on the knee of the leg in front. Repeat this exercise on the other leg.

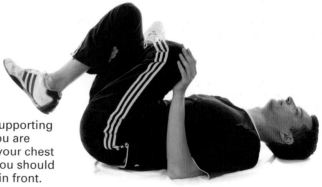

## Leaning Backward

This exercise focuses on developing the muscles in the lower back. Here you are performing a simple back exercise, where you lean backward in a slow and controlled action. If your muscles are tight in this region, you will find that you are unable to lean very far back, but over time you would expect to be able to increase this. Do not attempt this exercise if you have any back problems.

From a standing position, use your hands to support your back and then slowly lean backward. Continue as far as you can comfortably go.

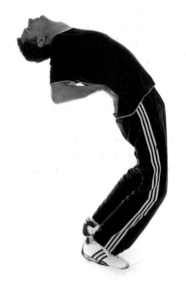

## Waist Twist

This is a simple refreshing exercise where you rotate the upper body in order to achieve a stretch in the spine. It can be useful as part of any warm-up or cool-down. Start with your feet hip-width apart and your arms resting by your sides. You then rotate your upper body around as far as you are able. Remember to repeat on the other side.

Stand with your feet hip-width apart and your arms by your side. Use your arms to help you twist the upper body. Go as far around as you are comfortable. Repeat on the other side.

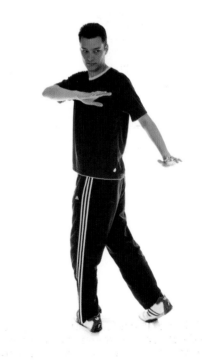

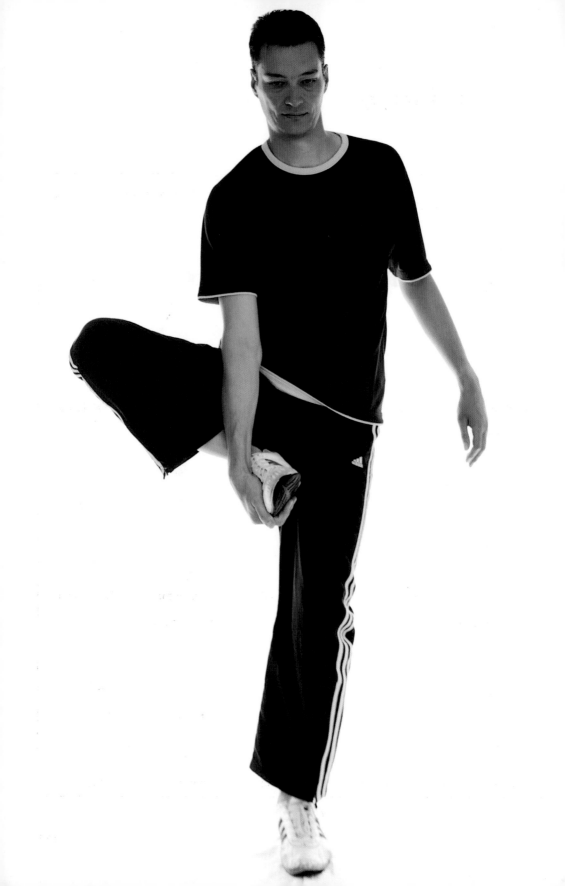

# 12 Balance

Balance: the ability to get into and maintain a state where the forces acting on the body are evenly distributed.

## Balance Exercises Summary

Standing exercises:

| | | | | |
|---|---|---|---|---|
| balls of the feet stand | tandem feet stand | heel stand | one-legged stand | on the ball of the foot |

Standing exercises:                                Walking exercises:

| | | | | |
|---|---|---|---|---|
| leg behind | leg in front | leg to the side | walking on toes | tandem walking |

Walking exercises:                                Movement exercises:

| | | | | |
|---|---|---|---|---|
| tandem backwards | heel walking | cross walking | jump | hop |

# ABOUT BALANCE

Balance is the ability to remain stable, due to the equilibrium between all of the forces acting on the body. Strength, vision, the function of the inner ear and coordination are all required in order to maintain a balanced position. It is possible to improve the ability to balance through regular practice. Balancing requires you to have a sense of your centre of gravity and continually to adjust the usage of your muscles and alignment. Simple techniques can be used to help maintain balance, such as focusing your gaze on a steady point, slightly bending at the knees, widening your base, or even starting by supporting yourself against a wall. When starting balance training, using a support structure in particular can help you to achieve a position while minimizing the risk of falling over.

There are three main sources of information collected by the brain in order to balance the body:

• Vestibular information from the ears. The ears contain a series of fluid-filled canals that contain small hair cells. It is these hair cells that detect movement of the fluid in the canals as the body moves around.
• Visual information through the eyes. The eyes tell the brain where the body is in relation to its surroundings.
• Proprioceptive information. The response to stimuli from the sensors in the joints and muscles. These sensors tell the brain where each part of the body is positioned and those in the skin will let the body know if it is in contact with something.

Symptoms such as travel sickness and finding balance more difficult in the dark may be caused by the improper interpretation of the vestibular and visual information. Disruption of any of these information sources can lead to dizziness and a loss of balance. This is believed to be caused by the brain trying to compensate for some lack of information from one of its three sources.

# BENEFITS OF TRAINING FOR BALANCE

Balance is a fundamental ability that can help to give you an edge in whatever sport or activity you are involved in. It can help you to reduce the chances of falling over in a variety of circumstances which can occur both inside and outside of a training environment:

• when somebody bumps into you
• when you trip on something
• when you are holding a difficult position
• when you are stretching to reach.

When balancing, it may look like you are really stable and not moving. In fact, your body will be constantly moving, even though the motion range and size may be small, in order to keep the body balanced. It is not possible to be perfectly still, as the body will continuously adjust to maintain its position. You can test this by standing on one leg and tuning in to how much work your body is doing in order to keep you in that position and to maintain the same centre of balance. Exercising to improve your balance will enable the brain to practise putting together all the information that it receives to achieve this. You may find that the first few times of trying balance exercises are difficult. Keep note of how you get on so that you can track your improvement over time.

# IMPROVING BALANCE

The balance exercises in this chapter can be performed with no special equipment, so that you are working with only your own body weight. When trying one of the exercises for the first time, do not use any additional weights. You should aim to choose exercises that you find challenging so that your body can work on developing your balance. Once a particular balance exercise becomes effortless, move onto something more difficult. You can increase the difficulty level, for example, by:

• closing your eyes
• increasing the range of motion
• increasing the speed of the movement part of the exercise
• adding free weights.

As with most types of exercises, the more you practise, the more improvement you will see. If you find it difficult to set aside time for practising, consider ways in which you could incorporate such activities into your daily routine. As you develop your balance, you may start to notice that you are becoming more aware of how your muscles work in order to help you to achieve more difficult balances. Strong muscles, particularly around the abdomen, should also help to improve your balance. So if you are working on developing your muscles through strength training, you may also find that your balance starts to improve as a natural consequence.

You may notice an improvement some time after you start practising. By deliberately exposing your body to exercises that challenge its balance, you encourage the brain to get better at interpreting the information it receives. You may sometimes experience off days where you feel particularly challenged. This could be caused by strain or tiredness. You should be aware of the sensation of imbalance and should work at the level at which that sensation begins. Do not work to the point at which you actually lose balance and fall over.

There are a number of sports and activities that can help to develop balance, for example:

• yoga
• dance
• martial arts
• gymnastics
• surfing.

Such activities are excellent for developing balance in a fun environment. Taking part in an activity that develops your balance should also help you to remain motivated with your training, as you will be able to see how others fare with the same exercises that you attempt.

The exercises in this chapter can help in developing your balance by training you towards holding the positions for increasing amounts of time. Some exercises can look deceptively easy. You may find that you are naturally good at balancing, or you may find that the opposite is true. If you find achieving any of the balancing positions difficult, it is better to focus on one of the preparatory steps instead until you are ready to progress through to the whole position. Focusing your gaze on a steady point in front of you should help you to balance. Watching other students wobbling in their position will tend also to make you feel unstable. Balancing with your eyes closed can be more difficult, so it is best to start with your eyes open before moving on. You can even use a wall to provide support initially, as this will help you to get into the position first and then work on the balance, rather than trying to do all things at once. Again, you should work towards holding the position for longer over time. It is better to hold a slightly easier position for a while than to hold a difficult position only momentarily. Further information can be found in Martin (2009), Brown (2003), Karter (2007), Craig and Taylor (2007) and Iyengar (1991).

If you wish to track the progress of your balance training, you could monitor it by using some simple indicators like those described overleaf. You can use this table to

**Measuring Improvement in Balance**

• Require a support structure, like a wall or a chair, to steady myself.
• Require both arms to steady myself.
• Require one arm to steady myself.
• Require no arms unless I lose balance during the exercise.
• Have my eyes closed and require both arms to steady myself.
• Have my eyes closed and require one arm to steady myself.
• Have my eyes closed and require no arms to steady myself.
• Have my eyes closed and require no arms to steady myself.
• Can increase the length of time that I hold the position.

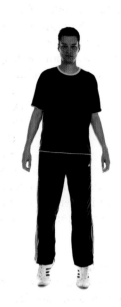

grade your ability to do the exercise and to monitor how you improve over time for the same exercises.

## SAFETY CONSIDERATIONS

You must ensure your training area is safe and that you train in such a way that you can be supported quickly if you become unsteady. For exercises that require movement in particular, you could train in a hall or other clear area. If you feel unsteady during an exercise, you could consider training near a corner or a wall so that you can quickly get support if you need it. You must immediately stop any exercise that makes you feel pain, dizziness, chest pain, fainting, or a change in your hearing.

## BALANCE EXERCISES

### Balls of the Feet Stand
This first exercise requires you to come up onto your toes while in a standing position. You should have both of your feet on the

Stand in a relaxed position with your feet one hip-width apart and firmly on the ground. Remain as still as possible. Slowly raise up onto the balls of your feet and focus on maintaining balance. Try to stay in this position for ten seconds. Repeat as required.

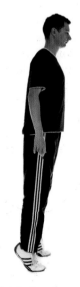

Side view of the balls of your feet stand.

ground, but only the balls of your feet will make contact with the floor. You may find it easier to stand in a corner, just away from the wall, so that you can quickly support yourself if you lose balance. Once you are in position, aim to stay as still as possible and not let the heels of your feet touch the ground at all. To make this exercise a little easier, bend your knees just a little. To make it more difficult, close your eyes. You may find you sway a little as your body tries to adjust to not having any information from your eyes to help it keep balanced. You may also feel your feet working hard at keeping you in position.

**Tandem Feet Stand**

This exercise is generally more difficult than standing on the balls of your feet, as it positions your feet heel to toe, one foot directly in front of the other. You may find you feel like swaying to either side whilst holding this position. Remember to repeat this exercise with the other foot in front. You may find it easier to stand in a corner, just away from the wall, so that you can quickly support yourself if you lose balance. Once you are in position, aim to stay as still as possible and not let the upper body move around too much. To make this exercise a little easier, bend your knees just a little. To make it more difficult, close your eyes. You may find that you sway a little as your body tries to adjust to not having any information from your eyes to help it keep balanced. You may also feel your feet working hard at keeping you in position.

**Heel Stand**

This exercise moves the weight of the body onto the heels of both of the feet. It looks easy, but is actually very difficult. Attempting this exercise will help you to understand how much adjustment and work your feet are normally doing for you

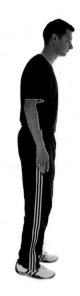

Step 1. Stand in a relaxed position with your feet one hip-width apart and firmly on the ground.

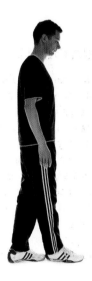

Step 2. Place your right foot directly in front of your left foot, such that the toes of your rear foot touch the heel of the front foot. Remember that your feet must be in line and that the heel of your front foot must touch the toes of your rear foot. Focus on maintaining balance and try to hold this position for ten seconds.

in the previous exercises. Here, you will find it difficult to hold the position more than momentarily because there is no reasonable way to make adjustments through your heels in order to maintain your balance. You are likely to feel a tendency to lose balance in either the forward or backward direction. You may find it easier to stand in a corner, just away from the wall, so that you can quickly support yourself if you lose balance. Once you are in position, aim to stay as still as possible and not let the balls of your feet touch the ground at all. To make this exercise a little easier, bend your knees just a little. To make it more difficult, close your eyes. You may find that you begin to sway a little as your body tries to adjust to not having any information from your eyes to help it keep balanced.

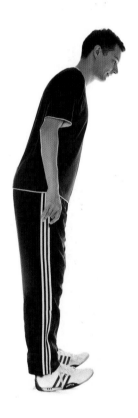

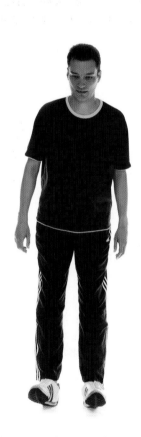

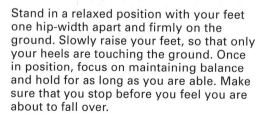

Stand in a relaxed position with your feet one hip-width apart and firmly on the ground. Slowly raise your feet, so that only your heels are touching the ground. Once in position, focus on maintaining balance and hold for as long as you are able. Make sure that you stop before you feel you are about to fall over.

Front view of the heel stand.

## One-Legged Stand

In this exercise, you start in the basic standing position, then raise one leg off the ground. Your raised foot should not touch your other leg. You should also focus on not letting your raised leg wobble around too much. Remember to repeat this exercise on the other side by raising the other leg. You may find it easier to stand in a corner, just away from the wall, so that you can quickly support yourself if you lose balance. Once you are in position, aim to stay as still as possible and not let your other foot touch the ground at all. To make this exercise a little easier, bend your knees just a little. To make it more difficult, close your eyes. You may find that you begin to sway a little as your body tries to adjust to not having any information from your eyes to help it to keep the body balanced. You may also feel your feet working hard at keeping you in position. This exercise can be made more difficult by increasing the height to which you raise your leg.

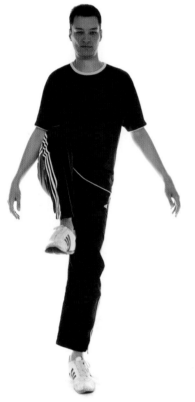

Stand in a relaxed position with your feet one hip-width apart and firmly on the ground. Rest your arms by your side. Slowly raise one leg off the floor. Do not let it touch your other leg. You can adjust the height of the raised leg to suit your ability level. Once in position, focus on maintaining balance and hold for ten seconds. Repeat on the other side.

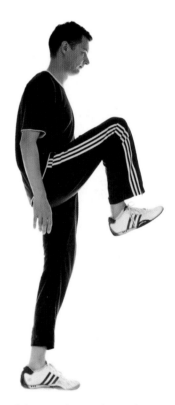

Side view of the one-legged stand.

### One-Legged Stand on the Ball of the Foot

This exercise builds on the previous 'balls of the feet stand'. Here you start in that position first, then slowly raise one of your legs. Your raised foot should not touch the other leg. You should also focus on not letting your raised leg wobble around too much. Remember to repeat this exercise on the other side by raising the other leg. You may find it easier to stand in a corner, just away from the wall, so that you can quickly support yourself if you lose balance. Once you are in position, aim to stay as still as possible and not let your other foot touch the ground at all. To make this exercise a little easier, bend your knees just a little. To make it more difficult, close your eyes. You may find that you begin to sway a little as your body tries to adjust to not having any information from the eyes to help keep it balanced. You may also feel your feet working hard at keeping you in position. This exercise can be made more difficult by increasing the height to which you raise your leg.

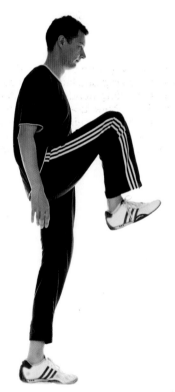

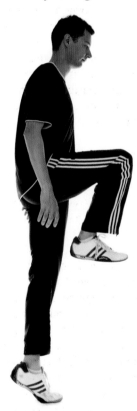

Step 1. Stand in a relaxed position with your feet one hip-width apart and firmly on the ground. Rest your arms by your side. Slowly raise one leg off the floor. Do not let it touch the other leg. You can adjust the height of the raised leg to suit your ability level. Once in position, focus on maintaining balance and hold for ten seconds.

Step 2. Now lift up your supporting leg so that only the ball of the foot is in contact with the ground. Once in position, focus on maintaining balance and hold for ten seconds.

## Holding One Leg Behind

This is quite a difficult exercise for both position and balance. You may want to practise this initially using a wall for supporting your leading hand. It stretches both the quadriceps and the lower back. To get into this position, start by standing with your feet hip-width apart, then raising one leg behind you so that you are in the standing quadriceps stretch position. From here, you should use one hand to hold the foot and help you to raise it higher off the ground. You no longer want the foot to be resting on your bottom. Raise it such that the toes try to point towards the ceiling. Try to keep your upper body as upright as possible. Do not make an active effort to lean forward. To make this exercise easier, bend the knee of the supporting leg. To make it more difficult, try holding this position with your eyes closed. The latter should only be attempted by advanced practitioners.

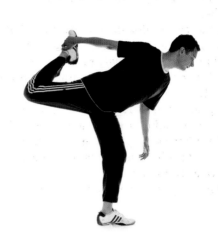

Start by standing with your feet hip-width apart, then raising one leg behind so that you are in the standing quadriceps stretch position. From here, use one hand to hold the foot and help you to raise it higher off the ground. You should continue to raise it such that the toes try to point towards the ceiling.

## Holding One Leg in Front

This is also quite a difficult exercise for both position and balance. You may want to practise this initially using a wall for supporting your back. It stretches the hamstrings in particular and requires strength. To get into this position, start by standing with your feet hip-width apart then raising one leg in front of you. From here, you should use one hand to hold the foot and help you to first straighten the raised leg. Once you are able to hold the straightened leg in this position, you could try lifting it higher. The leg must remain straight at all times. Try to keep your upper body as upright as possible. Do not make an active effort to lean forward or backward. To make this exercise easier, bend the knee of the supporting leg. To make it more difficult, try holding this position with your eyes closed. The latter should only be attempted by advanced practitioners. If you find this exercise too difficult, you could modify it so that you are lifting your knee to your chest rather than the entire straightened leg.

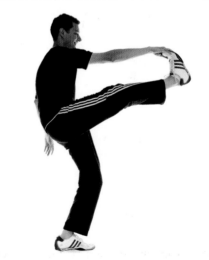

Start by standing with your feet hip-width apart and then raising one leg in front of you. From here you should use one hand to hold the foot and help you to first straighten the raised leg. Once you are able to hold the straightened leg in this position, then you could try lifting it higher.

## Holding One Leg to the Side

This is also quite a difficult exercise for both position and balance. You may wish to practise this initially using a wall for supporting your back. It stretches the hip adductors in particular and requires strength. To get into this position, start by standing with your feet hip-width apart then raising one leg with the knee out to the side of you. From here, you should use one hand to hold the foot and help you first to straighten the raised leg out to the side of your body. Once you are able to hold the straightened leg in this position, you could try lifting it higher. The leg must remain straight at all times. Try to keep your upper body as upright as possible. To make this exercise easier, bend the knee of the supporting leg. To make it more difficult, you could try holding this position with your eyes closed. The latter should only be attempted by advanced practitioners. If you find this exercise far too difficult, you could modify it so that you only go as far as Step 1 and focus on bringing the foot up as high as possible.

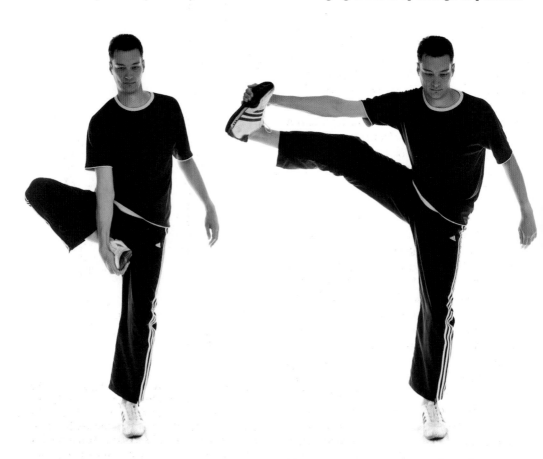

Step 1. Start by standing with your feet hip-width apart, then raising one leg with the knee out to the side.

Step 2. From this position, use one hand to hold the foot and help you to straighten the raised leg out to the side of your body. Once you are able to hold the straightened leg in this position, you could try lifting it higher.

## Walking on the Balls of the Feet

Start in the position where you are standing on the balls of your feet with your feet hip-width apart. Once you are balanced in this position, you should slowly take steps whilst keeping your feet in the same position, so that only the balls of your feet come into contact with the ground. Aim to keep your gaze forward and to walk in a straight line, slowly and controlled. This exercise is best performed in a hall or other clear area where you have enough space to walk ten steps. Ensure that there are no obstructions that would create a safety hazard. If you feel unbalanced, walk alongside a wall so that you can quickly support yourself if need be. To make this exercise easier, bend your knees just a little. To make it more difficult, close your eyes. You may find that you begin to sway a little as your body tries to adjust to not having any information from your eyes to help keep it balanced. You may also feel your feet working hard at keeping you in position.

## Walking Heel to Toe

Start in the position with your feet in tandem, standing heel to toe. Once you are balanced in this position, slowly take steps, walking heel to toe. Aim to keep your gaze forward and to walk in a straight line, slowly and controlled. This exercise is best performed in a hall or other clear area where you have enough space to walk ten steps. Ensure that there are no obstructions that would create a safety hazard. If you feel unbalanced, walk alongside a wall so that you can quickly support yourself if need be. To make this exercise easier, bend your knees just a little. To make it more difficult, close your eyes. You may find that you begin to sway a little as your body tries to adjust to not having any information from your eyes to help keep it balanced. You may also feel your feet working hard at keeping you in position.

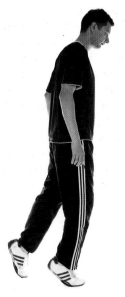

Stand in a relaxed position with your feet one hip-width apart and firmly on the ground. Slowly raise up onto the balls of your feet and focus on maintaining balance. Slowly step forward and continue to take ten steps and then rest.

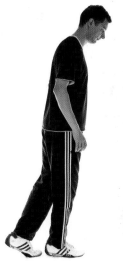
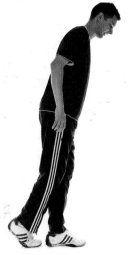

Step 1 (left). Stand in a relaxed position with your feet one hip-width apart and firmly on the ground. Slowly bring one foot forward and place it in front of the other. Remember that your feet must be in line and that the heel of your front foot must touch the toes of your rear foot. Focus on maintaining balance and try to hold this position for ten seconds.

Step 2 (right). Slowly step forward, walking heel to toe for ten steps, then rest.

## Walking Heel to Toe Backward

Start with your feet in the tandem position, where you are standing heel to toe. Once you are balanced in this position, slowly take steps going backward, walking heel to toe. Aim to keep your gaze forward and to walk in a straight line, slowly and controlled. This exercise is best performed in a hall or other clear area where you have enough space to walk ten steps. Ensure that there are no obstructions that would create a safety hazard. If you feel unbalanced, then you could try walking alongside a wall, so that you can quickly support yourself if need be. To make this exercise easier, bend your knees just a little. To make it more difficult, close your eyes. You may find that you begin to sway a little as your body tries to adjust to not having any information from your eyes to help keep it balanced. You may also feel your feet working hard at keeping you in position.

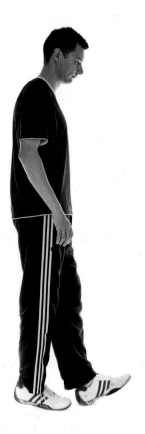 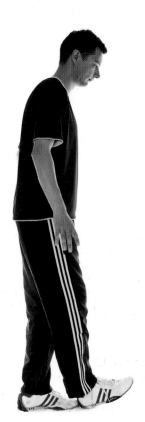

Step 1. Stand in a relaxed position with your feet one hip-width apart and firmly on the ground. Slowly bring one foot backward and place it behind the other. Remember that your feet must be in line and that the heel of your front foot must touch the toes of your rear foot. Focus on maintaining balance and try to hold this position for ten seconds.

Step 2. Slowly step backward, walking heel to toe for ten steps, then rest.

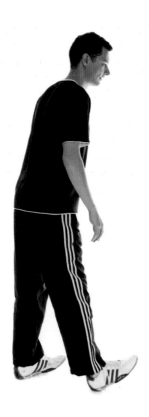 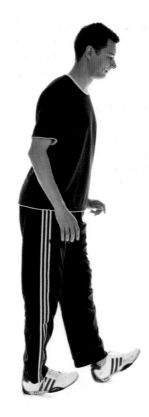

Step 1. Stand in a relaxed position with your feet one hip-width apart and firmly on the ground. Slowly raise your feet so that only your heels are touching the ground. Once in position, focus on maintaining balance and hold for as long as you are able. Make sure that you stop before you feel you are about to fall over.

Step 2. Slowly step forward, take ten steps and then rest.

## Walking on the Heels

Start in the position where you are standing on your heels with your feet hip-width apart. Once you are momentarily balanced in this position, slowly take steps whilst keeping your feet in the same position so that only the heels of your feet come into contact with the ground. Aim to keep your gaze forward and to walk in a straight line, slowly and controlled. This exercise is best performed in a hall or other clear area where you have enough space to walk ten steps. Ensure that there are no obstructions that would create a safety hazard. If you feel unbalanced, try walking alongside a wall so that you can quickly support yourself if need be. To make this exercise easier, bend your knees just a little. To make it more difficult, close your eyes. You may find that you begin to sway a little as your body tries to adjust to not having any information from your eyes to help it to balance. You may also feel your feet working hard at keeping you in position.

## Cross Walking

Start in the basic standing position, in which you are standing firmly with your feet hip-width apart. Once you are balanced in this position, slowly proceed to take steps. Your foot should come first in front, then to the side passing the rear foot, so that you are overall moving forward even though your feet move both forward and sideways with each step. Aim to keep your gaze forward and to walk in a straight line, slowly and controlled. This exercise is best performed in a hall or other clear area where you have enough space to walk ten steps. Ensure that there are no obstructions that would create a safety hazard. If you feel unbalanced, walk alongside a wall so that you can quickly support yourself if need be. To make this exercise easier, bend your kneed just a little. To make it more difficult, close your eyes. You may find that you begin to sway a little as your body tries to adjust to not having any information from your eyes to help it balanced. You may also feel your feet working hard at keeping you in position.

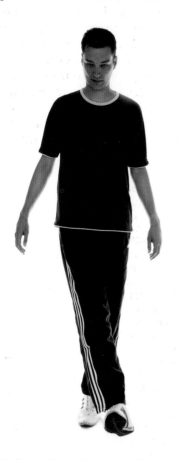

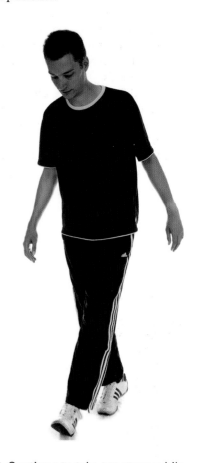

Step 1. Stand in a relaxed position with your feet one hip-width apart and firmly on the ground. Slowly step forward and let your leading foot pass in front of your other foot.

Step 2. Continue to take ten steps while crossing the feet in front of each other and then rest.

## Jump

Start in the basic standing position, with your feet firmly on the ground and one hip-width apart. Once you are balanced in this position, slowly proceed to take a jump. The balancing challenge is upon landing. Aim to keep your gaze forward. You could later increase the difficulty of this exercise by increasing either the height or the distance of the jump. You want to aim to land firmly on both of your feet at the same time and be in a balanced position, so that you or your arms do not wobble about on landing. You can check that you land on both of your feet at the same time by listening to the sound your feet make on landing. If you hear only one sound, you are landing with both feet at the same time. If you hear two sounds, your feet are contacting the ground at different times. This exercise is best performed in a hall or other clear area where you have enough space to perform the jump. Ensure that there are no obstructions that would create a safety hazard. If you feel unbalanced, then you could try jumping alongside a wall, so that you can quickly support yourself if need be.

## Hop

Start in the basic standing position, with your feet firmly on the ground and one hip-width apart. You then lift one leg up, so that your weight is completely supported on the other leg. Once you are balanced in this position, slowly take a hop. The balancing challenge is upon landing. Aim to keep your gaze forward. You could later increase the difficulty of this exercise by increasing either the height or the distance of the hop. Aim to land firmly on your foot and be in a balanced position, so that you or your arms do not wobble about on landing. Remember to repeat this exercise on the other side by raising your other leg. This exercise is best performed in a hall or other clear area where you have enough space to perform the hop. Ensure that there are no obstructions that would create a safety hazard. If you feel unbalanced, hop alongside a wall so that you can quickly support yourself if need be.

Stand in a relaxed position with your feet one hip-width apart and firmly on the ground. Slowly raise one leg off the floor. Do not let it touch your other leg. You can adjust the height of your raised leg to suit your ability level. Once in position, focus on maintaining balance and hold for ten seconds. Slowly perform a hop. Remember that you want to land firmly on your foot. Focus on maintaining balance and try to hold this position for ten seconds.

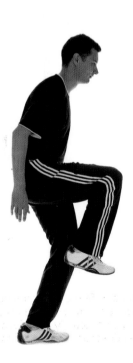

Stand in a relaxed position with your feet one hip-width apart and firmly on the ground. Slowly perform a jump. Remember that you want to aim to land firmly on both of feet, such that your feet touch the ground at the same time. Focus on maintaining balance and try to hold this position for ten seconds.

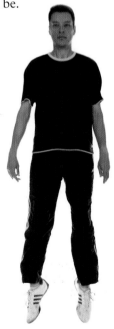

# 13    Quick Reference Guides

This chapter contains a visual summary of all of the exercises in this book. The idea is that it can be used as a reference during training. The summary tables are as follows:
• strength, strength endurance and power training exercises summary
• plyometrics training exercises summary
• stamina training exercises summary
• speed training exercises summary
• agility training exercises summary
• coordination training exercises summary
• posture training exercises summary
• flexibility training exercises summary
• balance training exercises summary

**Strength: the capacity to exert force. Strength endurance: the capacity of the muscles to withstand fatigue. Power: the capacity to generate large amounts of force in short periods of time.**

**Strength, Strength Endurance and Power Training Exercises Summary**

Ground exercises:

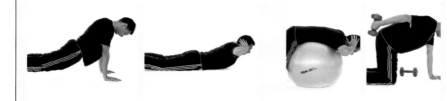

| press-up | back extension | Swiss Ball | triceps kick back | triceps push-up |

Ground exercises:                                                    Upper body exercises:

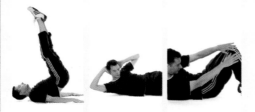

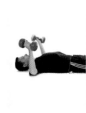

| reverse crunch | side crunch | opposites crunch | shrug | press | flye |

Upper body exercises:                          Standing exercises:

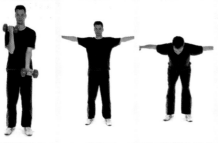

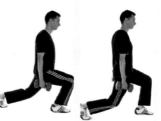

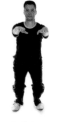

| curl | raise | bent-over raise | lunge | reverse lunge | squat |

*Plyometrics: the capacity to increase muscular forces using the stretch–shortening cycle.*

### Plyometric Exercises Summary

Improving jumping height:

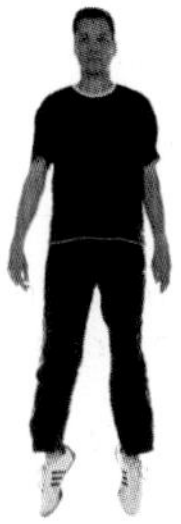

| small jumps | medium jumps | step jumps | knee tucks | jump squats |

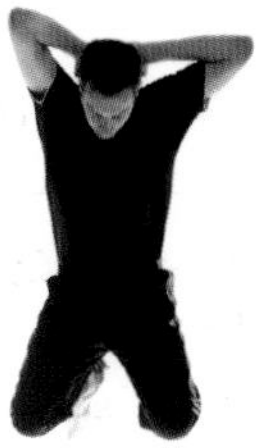

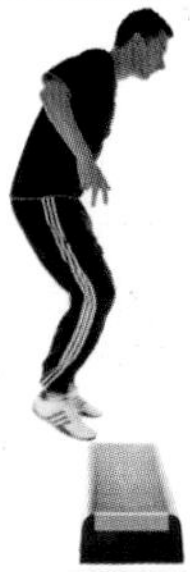

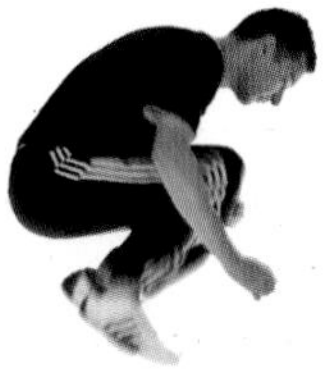

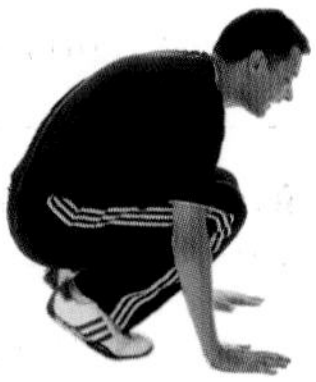

Improving distance:

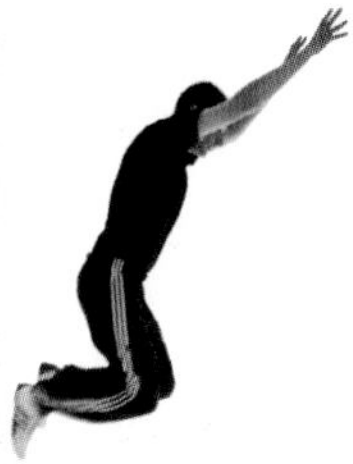

| jumping for distance | hopping for distance | bounding for distance |

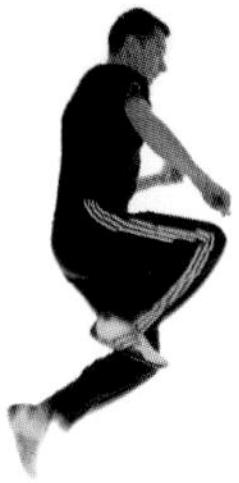

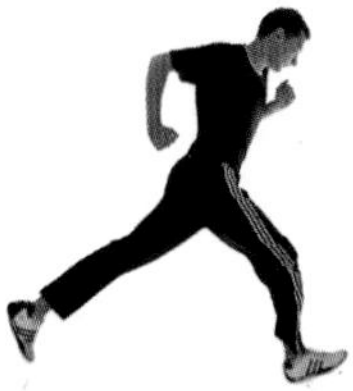

Conditioning the arms

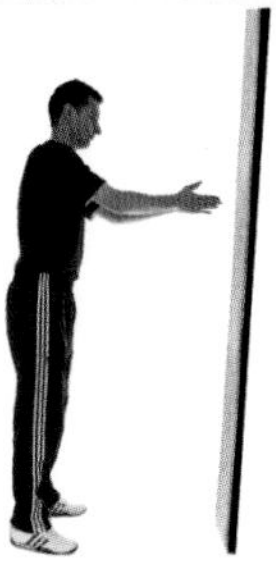

| vertical press-ups with a hand clap | horizontal press-ups with a hand clap |

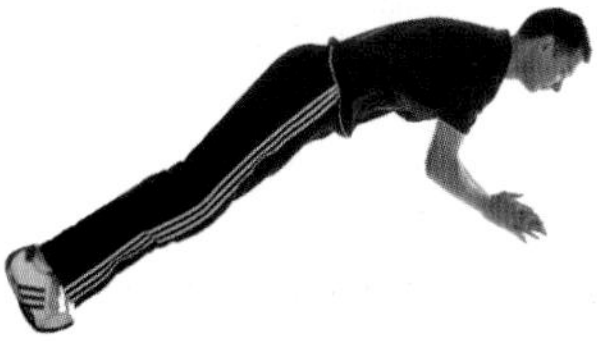

151

*Stamina: the capacity to sustain low-level aerobic work for a long period of time.*

### Stamina Exercises Summary

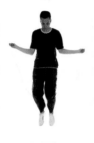

skipping

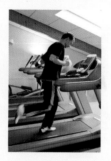

jogging

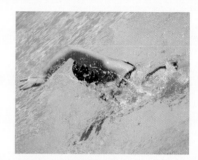

swimming

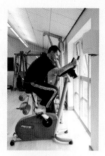

cycling

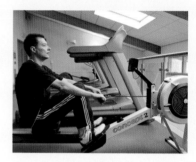

rowing

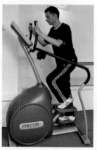

stair climbing

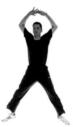

star jump and press-up combination

*Speed: the capacity to move the whole body or limbs quickly.*

## Speed Exercises Summary

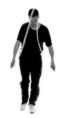

skipping with alternating feet

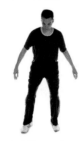

jumping in and out

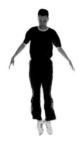

jumping side to side

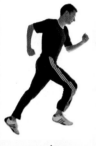

running

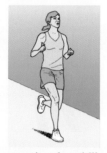

running downhill

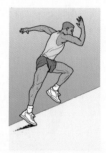

running uphill

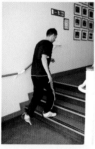

running up steps

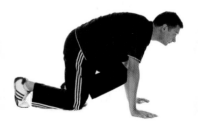

acceleration exercises

---

*Agility: the capacity to change direction rapidly.*

**Agility Exercises Summary**

On the spot:

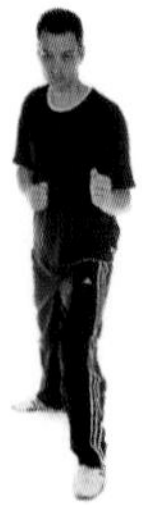

| | | |
|---|---|---|
| 90-degree turn | 180-degree turn | 270-degree turn |

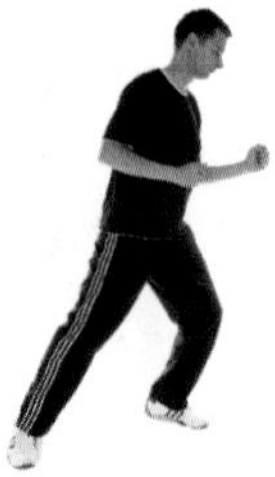

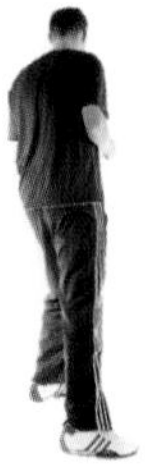

One step:

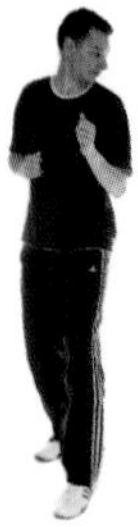

| | | |
|---|---|---|
| stepping forward with the leading leg and changing direction | pulling back foot and stepping backward | pulling back foot and stepping backward with change of direction |

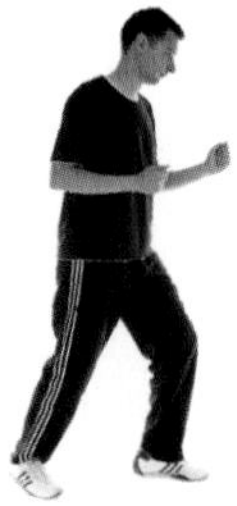

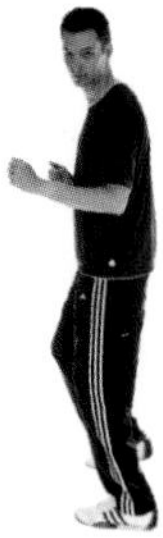

Multiple steps:

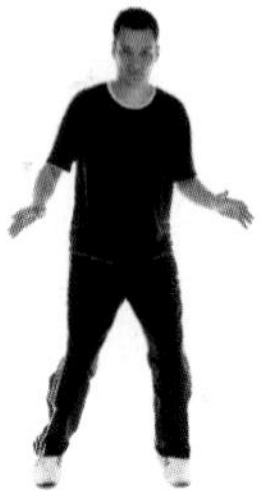

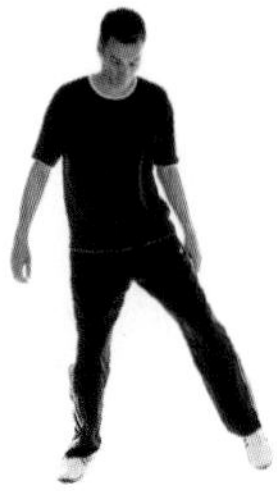

---

*Coordination: the ability to move body parts in a specific sequence.*

**Co-ordination Exercises Summary**

Using equipment:                                                                Arms:

| catching using one ball | catching using two balls | shuttlecock tapping | skipping | arms rotation |

Arms:                                                                           Legs:

| punching | upper-level block | mid-level block | low-level block | same side split jump |

Legs:          Arms and legs:

| opposite sides split jump | step and punch | step and block | step and opposite punch | step and opposite block |

155

**Posture: the capacity of certain core muscles to maintain efficient body alignment.**

### Posture Training Exercises Summary

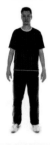 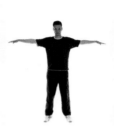 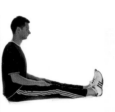 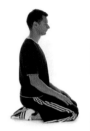

looking forward  standing with arms and legs out  sitting with the legs in front  sitting kneeling

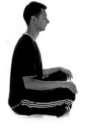 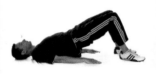 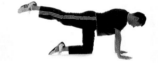

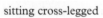

sitting cross-legged  bridging  dog

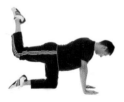 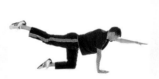 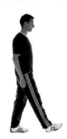

donkey  donkey with lifted arm  walking

156

*Flexibility: the range of movement around a joint or the amount of resistance to movement.*

**Flexibility Exercises Summary**

Arms:

Legs:

arm lifts in front     arm lifts to the side     triceps stretch     calves stretch

Legs:

standing hip adductors     sitting hip adductors     hamstring stretch     standing quadriceps

Legs:

Back:

lying quadriceps stretch     gluteals stretch     leaning backward     waist twist

**Balance:** *the ability to get into and maintain a state where the forces acting on the body are evenly distributed.*

## Balance Exercises Summary

Standing exercises:

| balls of the feet stand | tandem feet stand | heel stand | one-legged stand | on the ball of the foot |

Standing exercises:                                   Walking exercises:

| leg behind | leg in front | leg to the side | walking on toes | tandem walking |

Walking exercises:                                    Movement exercises:

| tandem backwards | heel walking | cross walking | jump | hop |

# Further Reading

Ackland, J., *The Complete Guide to Endurance Training* (A & C Black Publishers Ltd, 2007)

Bean, A., *The Complete Guide to Strength Training* (A & C Black Publishers Ltd, 2001)

Brown, C., *The Yoga Bible, The Definitive Guide to Yoga Postures* (Godsfield Press, 2003)

Brown, L. E. and Ferrigno, V., *Training for Speed, Agility and Quickness* (Human Kinetics Europe Ltd, 2005)

Buschmann, J., Pabst, K. and Bussman, H., *Co-ordination: A New Approach to Soccer Coaching* (Meyer and Meyer, 2001)

Bussell, D., *Pilates for Life: A Practical Introduction to the Core Programme* (Penguin, 2005)

Chu, D., *Jumping into Plyometrics* (Human Kinetics Europe Ltd, 1998)

Craig, C. and Taylor, M., *Get on It!: BOSU Balance Trainer Workouts for Core Strength and a Super Toned Body* (Ulysses Press, 2007)

Iyengar, B. K. S., *Light on Yoga* (Thorsons, 1991)

Kahn, J. and Biscontini, L., *Morning Cardio Workouts* (Human Kinetics Europe Ltd, 2006)

Karter, K., *Balance Training: Complete Stability Training for a Full Body Workout* (Ulysses Press, 2007)

Kielbaso, J., *Speed & Agility Revolution: Movement Training for Athletic Success* (Crew Press, 2005)

Lamb, D. R., *Physiology of Exercise* (Macmillan Publishing Company, 1984)

Lawrence, M., *The Complete Guide to Core Stability* (A & C Black Publishers Ltd, 2007)

Martin, A. P., *The Shotokan Karate Bible: Beginner to Black Belt* (A & C Black Publishers Ltd, 2007)

Martin, N. A., *Yoga for Flexibility, Strength and Balance: A Practical Structured Guide* (Crowood Press, 2009)

Norris, C. M., *The Complete Guide to Stretching* (A & C Black Publishers Ltd, 2001)

Radcliffe, J. C. and Farentinos, R. C., *High-powered Plyometrics* (Human Kinetics Europe Ltd, 1999)

Roberts, M., *The PHA Workout* (Dorling Kindersley Ltd, 2005)

Robinson, L., Fisher, H., Knox, J. and Thomson, G., *The Official Body Control Pilates Manual: The Ultimate Guide to the Pilates Method – For Fitness, Health, Sport and at Work* (Pan, 2002)

Smith, M., *High Performance Sprinting* (Crowood Press, 2005)

Ward, B. and Dintiman, G., *Sports Speed* (Human Kinetics Europe Ltd, 2003)

# Index

STRATHFIELD MUNICIPAL LIBRARY